ARKANA

WA-DO

Born in Vietnam, Dr Tran Vu Chi grew up in France and qualified in orthodox medicine in Paris, after studies in Tokyo embracing various aspects of traditional Japanese medicine including shiatsu and herbal medicine, as well as acupuncture and stress therapy. He has also studied a number of alternative medicines: homeopathy, osteopathy, oligotherapy and western herbal medicine. For some 15 years his work has been dedicated to the improvement of human health potential. He has a clinic in Paris where he treats patients with the system of Wa-Do which he has created. He has practised various forms of martial art, especially Aikido, and has experience in yoga and gymnastics.

Peter Megann holds an honours degree in modern languages and is an MA. He taught French language and literature until he retired. He is General Secretary of the British Aikido Federation and Aikido instructor at the Oxford University Aikido Club. Peter Megann holds 3 dan in Aikido (studying under Minoru Kanetsuka).

Wa-Do

Exercises for Health and Happiness

Tran Vu Chi

Translated from the French by Peter Megann

ARKANA

ARKANA

Published by the Penguin Group
27 Wrights Lane, London w8 5TZ, England
Penguin Books USA Inc., 375 Hudson Street, New York, New York 10014, USA
Penguin Books Australia Ltd, Ringwood, Victoria, Australia
Penguin Books Canada Ltd, 10 Alcorn Avenue, Toronto, Ontario, Canada M4V 3B2
Penguin Books (NZ) Ltd, 182–190 Wairau Road, Auckland 10, New Zealand

Penguin Books Ltd, Registered Offices: Harmondsworth, Middlesex, England

First published in France by Editions du Seuil 1988
This translation first published in Great Britain by Arkana 1990
10 9 8 7 6 5 4 3 2 1

French edition copyright © Editions du Seuil, 1988
This English translation copyright © Peter Megann, 1990
All rights reserved

Printed in Great Britain by Clays Ltd, St Ives plc
Filmset in 10½/12½ pt Ehrhardt

Contents

Preface

Everyone wants to be healthy and feel good, both in body and in mind. But why are these feelings of well-being so rare?

We live and express ourselves only through the things we possess. We boast: 'I have a husband, I have a wife, I have children, I have friends, I have a job, I have a car, I have a house ...' or we complain: 'I don't have time, I have problems, I have a pain ...' It is clear that we can find very little time simply to 'be'. 'To be or not to be?' is a question that is not asked! We simply no longer *are*. And there seems nothing we can do about it.

The answer is within our reach, however, and we should look for it inside ourselves, not through our possessions. 'To be' and 'to be well' are conditions that are attainable and can be achieved through physical means.

Let's experience the joy of exercising our bodies with a few simple movements, spontaneous and free from constraint – instinctive movements which we can rediscover. Let's forget our inhibitions and free that part of us which is essentially animal in its noblest and most innocent sense. Animals still possess this gift: for example, watch a cat walk along quite calmly, then suddenly leap to a great height as the restrained power of its body is suddenly released.

Why, then, should we try to acquire health, fitness or wonderful muscles by some miraculous external means? All we have to do is *feel health and fitness already within us*. We can experience a sense of well-being throughout our whole body – and it takes very little time. The aim of Wa-Do is to help us feel the power of life within us developing quietly but dynamically, without forcing anything. These exercises encourage natural healthy movements.

Of course, practising Wa-Do does not mean that we will never need to see a doctor, take medication or follow any prescribed treatment. But the very varied experiences I have had regarding health – orthodox medicine, alternative medicine, traditional medicine, Japanese anti-stress methods, martial arts, various gymnastic methods (both oriental and western) – have taught me that all too often we do not really know how to use our bodies and live in a healthy way. Physical education in schools is often inadequate, and in some countries it is counter-productive, despite the resources devoted to it. And suddenly taking up physical activity in mid-life can sometimes prove dangerous. In so-called civilized societies, we tend to neglect our bodies in favour of our intellectual activities, yet it is our bodies that make these activities possible. That is why I have created Wa-Do, on the foundations of orthodox medical science: first for myself and for those close to me, but also for my patients.

In everyday situations Wa-Do will help you find relief from discomfort, effectively, safely and sometimes instantly, by using simple, progressive movements, natural and easy to perform: the kind you have been searching for instinctively – *your own movements*. Other movements, equally simple, will strengthen your body and prevent the recurrence of health problems. Through the repetition of these movements, which you can practise *anywhere, any time, in a few moments, in any kind of clothing*, you will be able to rediscover the power of your body, which has been restricted for so long. You will experience, through your body, the pleasure of being alive instead of a feeling of 'having to put up with it', as is so often the case. As a result, you will feel the pleasure of knowing how to move your body naturally. You will be able to recognize the physical or sporting activities which suit it best, and feel your body opening out.

With its instinctive movements, Wa-Do is a little like good cooking, fine wine or making love! It is all a question of ingredients, personal preferences, instinct and common sense – plus a touch of originality. So let's start a healthy life: let's begin to make the most of things, try to form better habits and enjoy living. It *is* possible.

AN INTRODUCTION TO WA-DO

THE MYTHS

The myth of youth and speed

We live in an age of image and sound. To live quietly and contentedly is no longer considered acceptable. Our success and happiness depend on our appearance, for which we are prepared to make any sacrifice. We believe that youth is everything, that we should banish wrinkles and ugliness and become superfit. We fear that if we don't 'get the message' we will be pushed to one side and rejected. We think we don't have the right to look tired in today's world.

Young people pursue their active lives in bursts of frenetic energy, chasing the latest innovations and hungry for information, and saying: 'We must get the most out of life!' But the day is too short for them to do everything: there are just twenty-four hours in which to work, educate oneself, amuse oneself and sleep. We justify any means available to keep ourselves in trim: sports, weight-lifting, rejuvenation therapy and various cures, alternating blithely with cups of coffee, cigarettes, alcohol, tranquillizers and numerous other drugs and stimulants.

The myth of effort and suffering

Effort, then suffering, followed by a few short-lived pleasures, then more effort and more suffering. What a path to follow to reach fulfilment! In childhood we are made to sacrifice play – the expression of our dawning life – for the benefit of our precious studies. In school and university we are drawn into the same infernal conflicts: we learn about life by pushing ourselves harder and harder. We are made to feel that the more we know the more doors will open up for us – and that our future depends upon examination results. In every sphere of life and at every level of society, competition rules, dominating people's struggle for employment and their standard of living: a struggle for success and happiness.

In this marathon, stop for breath and you are out of the game. Take the sporting heroes we watch on our television screens: the tennis-player clutching his racket, the cyclist braced over his handlebars, the footballer struggling to keep up with the ball . . . Now there's health, we say. And we rush off to buy the same equipment, ready to follow in their footsteps. We say to ourselves: 'Where there's a will, there's a way.' And when it's our turn to perform, and it hurts, we consider that a good sign. We convince ourselves that we are on the right path. But is there only one path?

Effort and suffering, we soon discover, are not always crowned with success. We begin to have doubts: bitterness and resignation follow, then dejection and depression. We suddenly long for calm, for human tenderness and understanding. But isn't this the point from which we should have started? Isn't this path more likely to lead to stability, self-confidence and inner power? A fine wine does not improve if we shake it; it requires delicate handling and care. Are you beginning to understand?

I suggest that you look after your body as you would cherish a good wine. Become its attentive, understanding friend. Teach it to relearn the game; the movements it finds enjoyable and relaxing. Rediscover the right amount of effort your life requires, without getting tense and strained, without suffering. Simple enjoyment of living and peace within your body will set free your mind, which has been for so long inhibited by physical constraints. This state of well-being is sure to influence your relationship with the world around you and will allow you to confront life's hurdles with good humour.

The myth of good luck and good health

An increasing number of people are turning to astrology and fortune-tellers to predict their future health and success. Yet if they relied more on themselves and tried to understand themselves better, wouldn't they be better off in every way? When we are affected by an illness or an accident, we accuse fate of picking on us. These bouts of bad luck appear unjust; we cannot understand why they happen to us while others seem to be spared. And while modern medicine is so often able to help protect us from these blows, we expect it to come up with some miracle treatment in the form of a new vaccine, surgery, or a 'happy pill'. But have we really no role to play ourselves in the face of illness, or even before it? Illness arises from deep within our body; must we remain helpless victims and wait for illness to strike before we react? And does knowing the cause of an illness and the way to eradicate it mean that we understand how to promote good health? – It is not through the hidden face of the moon that we know its shining side. To discover the mechanism of an illness is certainly a good thing, but it would be better first to seek out the laws of good health and to find out if they can be directly applied to each individual.

After all, Newton was doing much the same when he reasoned that an apple which falls from a tree expresses the law of gravity. We are not all able to be scientific observers, of course, but certain laws which we search for are perhaps hidden by their very simplicity. Let's look at the way we behave, and think about the history of man. From earliest times man has been involved in a long process of continual adaptation to the conditions of life on earth, both during peace and in times of conflict, and throughout his evolution, each passage from one developmental stage to another has been marked by a crisis. A failure to take these crises into consideration leads to an over-simplified view of our history. Is it not a fact that the history of the earth, just as the universe, exists only through cataclysms?

We all have to learn to adapt to the conditions of our lives. When we don't adapt, we become ill. Is it the fault of our climate, our food, our work, where we live or of other people that we get ill? And where does fate fit in? Most of us are far too keen to take too much upon ourselves; trapped in a sedentary life, confined in the straitjacket of our body, we are weighed down with worries, duties and responsibilities. With life styles like these, isn't it rather fanciful to lay claim to good, long-lasting health? How can we possibly think and face life serenely under these conditions?

Let's learn to relax; in our mind, but above all in our body. Let's take an interest in it and train each of its functions to become more harmonious and lively. This is the way to understand the rules of health. There is nothing spectacular about this kind of programme. It is not a scientific discovery, but a discovery of oneself. Regular attention to our body's well-being can be seen as promoting the 'luck factor' of health to counteract the 'risk factor' of illness. Good luck and health can be within our grasp. Obviously the treatment of illness is a doctor's business, but our health is our individual responsibility.

REALITY

Let's stretch our tendons

Few people realize that it is through our tendons that we become tense. Everyone who recognizes this fact can get rid of nervous tension and relax in their everyday life. It need take only a few minutes, it is very simple and it can be done immediately. It's all a question of tendons.

Our muscles, which are made of an elastic fibre, can contract or relax. Our tendons, which are made of virtually inextensible fibres, stretch or slacken like a rope. Muscles respond to variations in length: tendons respond to varying degrees of tension. Muscles, which receive a good supply of blood, can recover more quickly than tendons, which are less well provided with blood vessels. For example, tendons which get strained during sport are more difficult to treat than muscular cramps. Repeated stress to muscles can cause deterioration in tendons. When we live a sedentary life, sitting for hours at a time (or standing), our body suffers because its tendons are being misused by a fixed posture or repetitive movements.

So let's learn to relax our tendons! This is a simple reflex bodily action that we should learn and use as often as possible. *This is the first exercise for well-*

being. If we use it, our whole nervous system will benefit and our performance throughout the day will improve.

How should we go about it? By repeating simple movements to and fro without any jerks or jolts; these small stretching and relaxing movements will allow the blood to circulate around the tendons. Continue to practise these movements in a natural, relaxed way; never force the stretching or prolong it so as to cause excessive tendon fatigue, for this will lead to muscle contraction which can sometimes take time to put right and is harmful to the whole nervous system.

Stretch gently. Let go gently. Rediscover the pleasure of relaxation.

Let's relax our muscles

We spend a great part of our lives tensed up: jaws clenched, breathing tightly, our backs slightly bent and our shoulders rounded. We seem to be involved in an endless struggle. We feel that we earn our living by the sweat of our brow, and we don't find it easy, having to be constantly on the alert and ready to react. But our sedentary lives mean that most of us are suffering from muscular atrophy. Sometimes just staying in one position becomes painful — we get cramps and aches, and whether they are transitory or permanent, they take all the pleasure out of life and seriously impair the synchronization of our movements. How can we get rid of this problem and help ourselves to relax?

Unlike sprinters or jumpers, whose exertions are of only short duration, most of us have professional, domestic and social lives which continue throughout the day. What we are asking from our atrophied muscles is nothing short of an endurance test for which we have no training. Some people find they can't cope and retire from this obstacle course exhausted and drained, disappointed, but also relieved. What has happened to them is quite understandable, however: they have failed to meet the demands of a gruelling life style because they have not been prepared for it. Our body, like our mind, needs regular, suitable training without overdoing it.

To be fresh and in good condition, a muscle must remain responsive to the variations in the length of its fibres. When we are re-educating our muscles, it must be done in a well-regulated way – and in a relaxed fashion, without the use of force. Any movement that requires force and power is always accompanied by a rapid accumulation of lactic acid in the muscle, and by fatigue. Relaxed movement, even though maintained for some time, does not have these results. Our muscles require natural, basic movements. Be gentle with them, and stay relaxed.

Let's loosen up

Some of us enjoy making our finger, neck or back joints crack! We may feel stiff, 'knotted up' and cramped; then 'crack' – with one or two conscious or unconscious movements, we suddenly feel loose and free. What has happened? Certainly nothing serious, for our bones are not cracked or broken – our joints have simply moved and made themselves more comfortable.

Many of us live with our tendons in a state of tension and our muscles in a state of contraction, so it's hardly surprising that our joints suffer. Ligaments that link them with the articular cartilage surrounding them tend to contract and harden with time. Our joints are permanently under pressure, and this can, in the long run, destroy the joints themselves. We gradually get used to the threat of chronic arthritis. But why allow ourselves to be trapped into letting this happen? We must slow down the process of premature ageing – by opening out and expanding our physical range.

This is what we are instinctively trying to do when we make our bones crack. But is it really necessary to become a disjointed puppet to avoid arthritis? (And it can involve a risk of injuring our ligaments and articular cartilages, or even of trapping a passing nerve and causing neuralgia.)

Let's take care of ourselves and avoid sudden or jerky movements. The ligament structure around a joint is made up of fibres that cannot stretch very much (it is these which can tear or cause sprains or dislocations when we have a fall), so we have to stretch these fibres gently, without damaging them. This is the path to suppleness. Do away with stiff joints. Loosen yourself up!

Let's give ourselves air

'Ah, a nice breath of fresh air!' is an everyday remark which could be called a cry from the lungs. Living as we do, closed in and crowded together, we cannot really breathe properly any more – or, at least, we do not breathe enough. Imperceptibly, we are asphyxiating in a limited supply of air. To forget to breathe properly is crazy; it is like forgetting how to live. It's possible for us to eat and drink nothing for several days without dying, but we can go without breathing for only about three minutes – no more. From the moment we are born, air is our essential sustenance, but, despite this, we hardly breathe properly at all. Have we too much on our minds, or are we too busy to bother about something so essential?

All our cells need oxygen, but the nerve cells need it most of all. Our whole nervous system, which controls our thinking, actions, digestion and excretion, is linked to life by this umbilical cord of breath. Even the slightest neglect can result in a number of bodily malfunctions.

Let's put matters right quickly and allow our lungs to play their proper role. They are like balloons which we can inflate or deflate at will, and they need to be used properly. So let's give them air. This will help us to live much healthier lives, and our muscles, tendons, joints and all our organs will benefit. Each time we inhale air into our lungs, it's as if we are born afresh!

Let's get our blood moving

A strong heart and a good circulation are generally regarded as the two winning cards in the game of health, while a heart attack is top of the list in all categories of fatal illness. 'Stop smoking!' 'Cut down the cholesterol!' the media warn repeatedly. But even if we wage a campaign against these unhealthy habits, we find that we are still attacked by their allies, stress and lack of exercise, both of which can increase the risk of a heart attack. And if our body is already suffering from high blood-pressure, obesity or diabetes, what can we do?

Numerous statistical studies have shown that a reasonable programme of physical exercise, combined with control in the consumption of tobacco and animal fats, offers many advantages: for example, an increase in the level of 'good cholesterol' in the blood, a lowering of blood-pressure, and the development of new circulatory networks. But what kind of exercise is best for us to take?

A word of warning here: only gentle, systematic exercising is recommended – any kind of intensive, brutal training should be banned. This is particularly true for those in sedentary occupations who are subject to stress: such training would increase their risk of a heart attack. Exercising the large muscular masses of our bodies will pump a large volume of blood and help the heart to work. So it is more useful to exercise our legs than our biceps. And a rhythmical kind of exercise, without jerky movements, will help to achieve a well-functioning circulation.

Our obsession with heart attacks, however, must not make us forget the other major risks connected with the circulation: a cerebro-vascular accident (or 'stroke') – often with the dramatic results of hemiplegia – and arteritis (inflammation of the arteries) in the legs, which can lead to gangrene. The circulation of the blood supplies all the tissues of the body, and when an area is badly supplied, the functions of the nearest organs are affected. It is no use

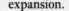

expansion.

After air, it is water that gives life.

To be fertile, the earth needs water.

To be healthy, the body needs good circulation of the blood.

So . . . improve it!

Let's take the pressure off

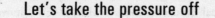

over-excitement. Even as we enjoy our coffee break, we cannot stop ourselves thinking about what we still have to do and how we shall cope with unforeseen problems. What an obstacle course!

Enough of this! Calm down. Stop thinking about whatever it is that's bothering you. Take the pressure off. Step back and size up the situation – the earth won't stop turning if you relax. Give your nerves a treat – reduce their overload.

The state of our nervous system reflects the pressure that we are under. But what can we do about it? First we must mobilize the blood supply to our tendons, muscles and joints, to reduce stagnation. Then we will begin to feel a reduction of nervous pressure in these areas. Do the same with your neck, to the sympathetic nervous system which controls the brain's circulation. Next, the region of your solar plexus, which controls the functions of the organs in the upper part of your abdomen. After that, move on to the other parts of the body.

We should learn to understand our hormonal system, which functions in harmony with our nervous system. The hormones are capable of modulating the effects of the nervous system on the body, both in intensity and in quality. The thyroid gland, in the neck, and the suprarenal glands, in the abdomen, can benefit from specific attention.

Every function of the body, whether organic or superior (such as intelligence), is under the control of the nervous system and the hormonal system. Without them our body would be like a wonderful machine with no current to make it run. Birth, growth, movement, thought – all life's actions are under their control. It is a perfect adaptation system, given to us when we are born, and it also allows us to communicate with the life around us. Without a sound nervous system, preserved by a good blood supply, any bodily development, sense of balance or recovery would be unlikely, nor would the functions it controls be shielded from deficiency. Indeed, without a sound nervous system our body could even grow old prematurely. To take the pressure off is an act of faith: faith in life. Let's take the pressure off.

THE MIRACLE

On the threshold of the third millennium, we enjoy a multitude of discoveries produced by the human genius. There is not a corner of the universe into which our intelligence has not penetrated – the earth, outer space, time . . . We pride ourselves on the explosion of knowledge in communication technology. We know how to control nuclear energy, how to create artificial intelligence, how to master everything, including the creation of human life. Where will it all end? A small voice within us sometimes reminds us of a very simple truth: '*The first wonder of the world is our own body.*'

When we feel good, worries and problems seem smaller and easier to solve. But when we are 'under the weather', everything soon becomes intolerable, as if the whole world were in league against us. We feel that the good things in life are slipping between our fingers. We can be feeling perfectly happy, then someone comes along and upsets us and our happiness disappears. Similarly, when we are unwell, we seem to stop living and are unable to appreciate the wonderful world around us. It's then that we realize that our body governs everything. Physical upsets can affect our whole attitude to life. For example, a simple back pain (a common complaint) affects our posture and will sometimes make us so hunched up that our lungs cannot expand properly. We start to miss the oxygen that our cells need, and digestive disorders begin to appear. If the nerves in our neck and shoulders become irritated, resulting in prolonged stiffness, we experience bouts of tiredness, 'pins and needles' in the arms and hands, and a heavy feeling in the head because of poor circulation. Indigestion creates abdominal tension, which restricts the movement of the diaphragm and may lead to the onset of a cold.

We can find endless examples to prove that our body works as an indivisible unity, that an upset in one of its functions inevitably affects others. We can put up with certain disorders, while others seriously interfere with our daily lives. We usually lay the blame, unjustly, on one particular organ – 'I've got stomach ache,' 'My nerves are on edge,' 'I can't breathe properly' – but it is our whole body that is ill and needs attention; its entire physiological balance is affected, even though it is only one organ that is causing discomfort.

To allow this state of affairs to continue can only harm us in the long run: as time goes on we shall succumb imperceptibly to other chronic, serious or degenerative illnesses. Are we just going to sit there and let this happen? Restoring the harmonious performance of each of the functions that have been upset seems to be the only logical solution for preserving or improving our health, and the restoration of each function will inevitably have an effect on the others. So let's create a 'chain of friendship' between our organs. Let's establish a real, conscious, friendly communication with our body and its organic functions. Let's reconnect the essential links of our interior world and forget about searching for a happiness that is light years away. 'Happiness is within you' – who can doubt it? But the first step to achieving it should be to start taking good care of our body. Let's rediscover our real body and its hidden potential. It cannot live without air, without water, or without an influx of life, and to these three vital needs correspond three functions which are ineffectively used by most people in their everyday lives. *The three prime laws of life and health are: breathing, the circulation of the blood, and the nervous and hormonal system.*

First of all, we must maintain and train these three functions, to reanimate and develop the colossal energy which lies within us. We must live in direct contact with our bodies.

The three gifts of vitality, joy and youthfulness are within us. Our civilization may well develop inexhaustible wealth in the future, but man will have to learn to live more from within if he is to survive. We can do it. It is simple – much simpler than mastering mathematics or driving a car in the rush hour! All it needs is a grain of common sense and a little courage to acquire this new reflex. It could even be quite fun, and we can do it any time. We already have the coffee-drinking reflex, and the cigarette-smoking reflex – why not a Wa-Do reflex? It's simple, it's enjoyable and it's always beneficial.

1 The nervous system

Life is founded on the nervous system, which originates in the brain and spreads down through the spinal canal, animating the arms, supporting the chest, abdomen and the lumbar area, and finally reaching the legs and feet.

We have only to observe the development of a baby to understand how this process works. In the beginning a baby only moves its head and motivates its features. Gradually it can move its arms and its fingers. Later it can sit up and use its legs. Finally it can stand up unaided and walk.

The nervous system is composed of two parts: the unconscious, which we can call the *basic nervous system*, and the conscious, which we can call the *complementary nervous system*. Of these the conscious is by far the most important. It controls our movements and the functioning of our organs in response to our vital needs (breathing, the circulation of the blood, the regulation of temperature, the intake and digestion of food and the elimination of waste products).

A *The basic nervous system*

● *the autonomic nervous system* regulates our inner activities (circulation of the blood, respiration, digestion, etc.) both in periods of activity and at rest
● *the involuntary nervous system* regulates our outer activity
● *the hormonal system* allows our body to speed up or slow down any form of activity, inner or outer.

B *The complementary nervous system*

This enables us to develop the life which is within us and gives us freedom of thought and action. It is composed of two parts:

● *the voluntary system*, which allows us to bring to conclusion the movements we wish to make

● *the executive system*, which allows us to gather information from our inner and outer worlds and to act upon it.

1 primary brain (hypothalamus) controls vital functions and innate behaviour
2 centre of emotions and memory
3 thinking, recording and decision-making area

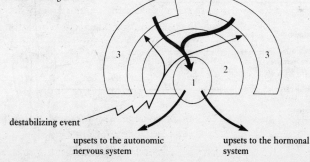

destabilizing event

upsets to the autonomic nervous system

upsets to the hormonal system

(i) Unconscious reactions of the basic nervous system to a stressful situation

(ii)   *Disorders of the autonomic nervous system*

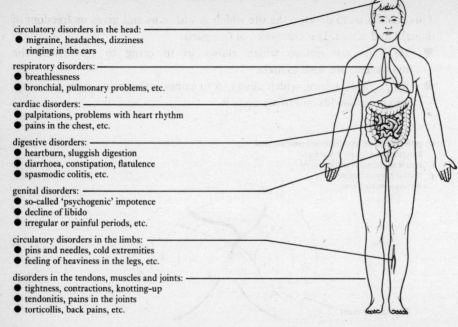

circulatory disorders in the head:
- migraine, headaches, dizziness
  ringing in the ears

respiratory disorders:
- breathlessness
- bronchial, pulmonary problems, etc.

cardiac disorders:
- palpitations, problems with heart rhythm
- pains in the chest, etc.

digestive disorders:
- heartburn, sluggish digestion
- diarrhoea, constipation, flatulence
- spasmodic colitis, etc.

genital disorders:
- so-called 'psychogenic' impotence
- decline of libido
- irregular or painful periods, etc.

circulatory disorders in the limbs:
- pins and needles, cold extremities
- feeling of heaviness in the legs, etc.

disorders in the tendons, muscles and joints:
- tightness, contractions, knotting-up
- tendonitis, pains in the joints
- torticollis, back pains, etc.

Plan of action
- action specific to each of the functions (see the following pages).

(iii)   *Problems of the hormonal system*

malfunction of the thyroid gland: ──────────
- fall in the secretion of thyroid hormones
- slowing down of physical and mental functions

malfunction of the adrenal gland (outer part: the cortex): ──────
- increase in the level of cortisol in the blood causes a lowering of the body's immune system (leading to infections and inflammations)
- problems with the metabolism of sugar, fats, water
- risk of high blood-pressure, obesity, diabetes

problems with the adrenal gland (central part: the medulla):
- tendency to high blood-pressure (so-called essential hypertension)
- risk of disease of the kidneys, heart and cerebral circulation

increase in blood-pressure

adrenal gland
kidney

Plan of action
- *in the neck:*
  encourage better circulation to the thyroid gland
- *in the upper part of the lumbar region:*
  improve the blood supply to the autonomic nervous pathways controlling the regions of the kidneys and the adrenal glands.

(iv) A 'voluntary' movement can arise only from 'involuntary' phenomena

Let's take a very ordinary example, observing the developing sequence of events from the decision to make a movement to its completion.

Good circulation within the brain	1	*I want an apple.*	decision to make the movement	= motor centre in action
	2	*Am I really hungry?*	vital need	= hypothalamus in action
	3	*Is it edible?*	emotional memory	= limbic system of the brain in action
	4	*Have I got time?*	reflection	= neocortex hemisphere in action
Control of involuntary actions (tendons, muscles, joints) tone, position, synchronization	5	*I put down the book I am holding and I start to move.*	programme of simple, elementary movements	= premotor centre in action
	6	*I do not hesitate. I do not tremble.*	synchronizing the contraction and relaxation of muscles	= central grey matter in action
	7	*My hand attains its goal without loss of balance.*	co-ordination of time/space, and balance	= cerebellum and vestibular formation in action
	8	*Satisfactory rhythm of my movement.*	speeding up or slowing down of command	= reticular formation in action
Equilibrium of the central and autonomic nervous systems	9	*My respiration, my circulation are as they should be and do not interrupt my action.*	autonomic and central nervous systems	= respiration and adrenalin hormone in action
	10	*I take hold of the apple.*	command to the hand to contract	= motor nerves

If the involuntary performers are in any way deficient, nervous expenditure will increase and the harmony and efficiency of the movement will be impaired.

2 Respiration

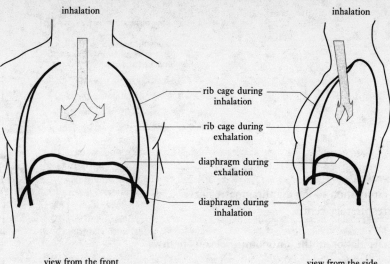

view from the front

view from the side

The diaphragm works a little like an umbrella, opening when air goes into the lungs and closing when the air goes out. During inhalation it pushes the abdominal organs downwards; on exhalation it pulls them upwards. It acts like a piston.

The diaphragm muscle divides the trunk into two compartments: the chest and the abdomen. It is attached to the ribs and the lumbar vertebrae and plays an essential role in the circulation of the blood, drawing the venous blood towards the heart during inhalation, thus helping it to perform properly.

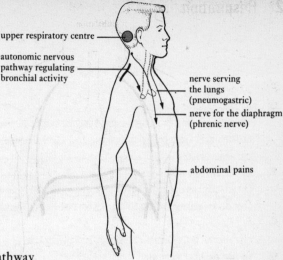

upper respiratory centre

autonomic nervous
pathway regulating
bronchial activity

nerve serving
the lungs
(pneumogastric)

nerve for the diaphragm
(phrenic nerve)

abdominal pains

Plan of action

- *at the back of the neck:*
  encourage better circulation to the diaphragmatic nerve,
  and to the upper respiratory centre
- *at the top of the back:*
  encourage better circulation to the autonomic nervous pathway
- *at the throat and on the chest:*
  encourage better circulation to the pneumogastric nerve serving the lungs
- *in the abdomen:*
  eliminate tension in the abdominal organs
- *around the rib cage:*
  improve the functioning of the respiratory muscles, their tendons, and the articulation of the rib cage
- *by direct action:*
  stimulate the diaphragm and pelvis, the trachea and bronchi, and the alveoli (small air sacs in the lungs).

3   The circulation of the blood

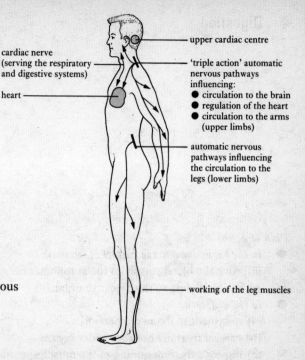

cardiac nerve
(serving the respiratory
and digestive systems)

heart

upper cardiac centre

'triple action' automatic
nervous pathways
influencing:
● circulation to the brain
● regulation of the heart
● circulation to the arms
  (upper limbs)

automatic nervous
pathways influencing
the circulation to the
legs (lower limbs)

working of the leg muscles

Plan of action
● *at the back of the neck:*
  encourage better circulation to the 'triple action'
  autonomic nervous pathways, and to the upper
  cardiac centre
● *in the throat and chest:*
  (a) encourage better circulation to the cardiac nerve
  (b) do exercises akin to an 'external heart massage'
● *in the abdomen:*
  eliminate tension in the abdominal organs
● *in the lumbar region:*
  (a) encourage better circulation to the autonomic nervous
  pathways, resulting in better circulation in the legs
  (b) improve the functioning of the muscles, tendons
  and joints in the areas of the back concerned
● *by direct action:*
  (a) deep inhalation, which improves the return of blood to the heart and helps the heart in its work
  (b) rhythmical working of the leg muscles, which has the same effect, and tends to normalize blood-
  pressure (in cases of high blood-pressure).

4 Digestion

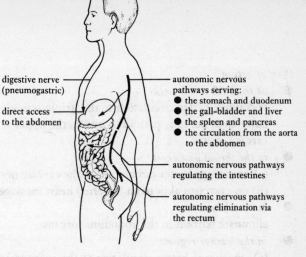

digestive nerve
(pneumogastric)

direct access
to the abdomen

autonomic nervous
pathways serving:
- the stomach and duodenum
- the gall-bladder and liver
- the spleen and pancreas
- the circulation from the aorta
  to the abdomen

autonomic nervous pathways
regulating the intestines

autonomic nervous pathways
regulating elimination via
the rectum

Plan of action
- *in the back, down to the buttocks (sacrum):*
  improve the blood supply to the autonomic nervous
  pathways leading to the digestive organs
- *in the abdomen:*
  (a) treatment to the nerve networks
  (b) careful treatment of the tender organs
  (c) improve the functioning of the muscles, tendons and joints of the back
- *by direct action:*
  deep breathing, which brings about a return of venous blood from the digestive system, via the liver, to the heart, and also induces healthy functioning of the intestines.

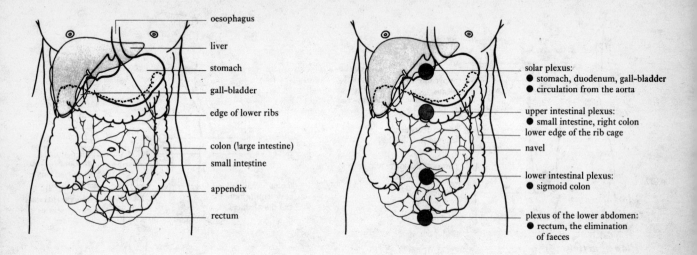

Digestive organs

oesophagus
liver
stomach
gall-bladder
edge of lower ribs
colon (large intestine)
small intestine
appendix
rectum

Nerve networks (plexuses)

solar plexus:
● stomach, duodenum, gall-bladder
● circulation from the aorta

upper intestinal plexus:
● small intestine, right colon
lower edge of the rib cage
navel

lower intestinal plexus:
● sigmoid colon

plexus of the lower abdomen:
● rectum, the elimination
 of faeces

5 The elimination of urine

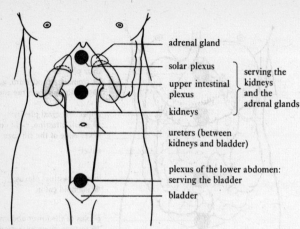

adrenal gland

solar plexus

upper intestinal plexus

kidneys

} serving the kidneys and the adrenal glands

ureters (between kidneys and bladder)

plexus of the lower abdomen: serving the bladder

bladder

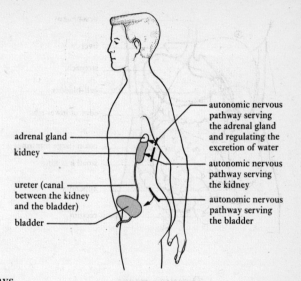

adrenal gland

kidney

ureter (canal between the kidney and the bladder)

bladder

autonomic nervous pathway serving the adrenal gland and regulating the excretion of water

autonomic nervous pathway serving the kidney

autonomic nervous pathway serving the bladder

Plan of action

- *just above the lumbar region:*
  improve the circulation to the autonomic nervous pathways
- *at the sacrum* (*top part of the pelvis*):
  the same treatment
- *in the abdomen:*
  (a) treatment of the solar plexus and upper intestinal plexus to improve the functioning of the kidneys
  (b) treatment to the plexus of the lower abdomen to improve the functioning of the bladder.

6 Genital function

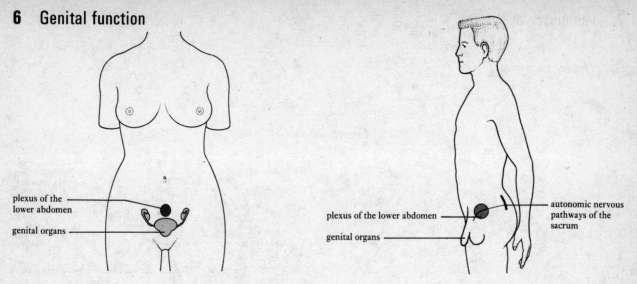

plexus of the
lower abdomen

genital organs

plexus of the lower abdomen

genital organs

autonomic nervous
pathways of the
sacrum

Plan of action
- *at the sacrum:*
  improve the circulation
- *in the abdomen:*
  improve the circulation.

7   The muscular system

(*i*)   *The neck muscles*

Superficial muscles

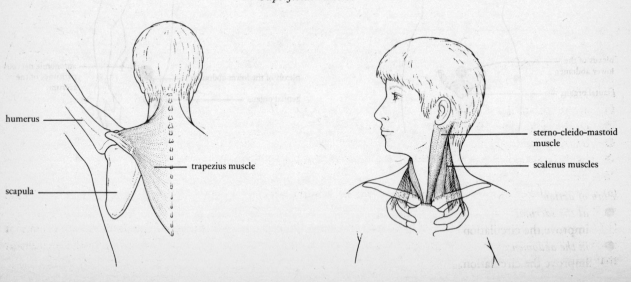

humerus

trapezius muscle

scapula

sterno–cleido–mastoid muscle

scalenus muscles

Deep muscles

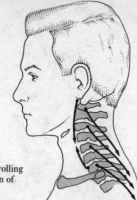

muscles controlling
the inclination of
the vertebrae

muscles controlling the
inclination of the head

Plan of action
- at the base of the skull (occiput)
- on the cervical vertebrae
- on the shoulder-blade
- by different positioning of the head, the neck, the back, and the arms.

Note well:

(a) a large number of muscles descend from the neck to the back: treatment to the back has repercussions in the neck and vice versa

(b) the small muscles beneath the base of the skull serve the continual adjustment of the head and are often in a state of permanent contraction, preventing the proper supply of blood to the nerves issuing from the medulla at that point.

(*ii*) *The muscles of the back*

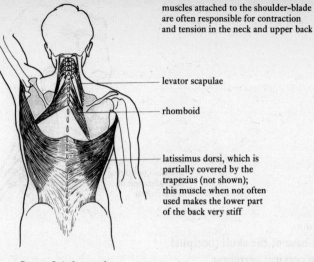

muscles attached to the shoulder-blade
are often responsible for contraction
and tension in the neck and upper back

— levator scapulae

— rhomboid

— latissimus dorsi, which is
partially covered by the
trapezius (not shown);
this muscle when not often
used makes the lower part
of the back very stiff

Superficial muscles

Note that the muscles of the back of the neck finish at the top of the back – pain in this area can be due to contractions and tension in the back of the neck.

The muscles of the lumbar region mostly start from the top of the back: tensions higher up the back can thus have repercussions in the lumbar area. Moreover, the transverse abdominal muscle is attached to the lumbar vertebrae and serves as a 'muscular belt': obesity stretches it and can cause pain in the lumbar area. A certain number of muscles are attached to the pelvis, where they can cause pain.

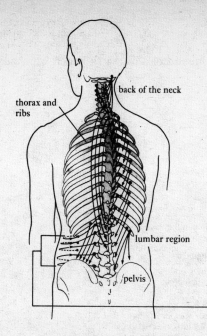

back of the neck

thorax and
ribs

lumbar region

pelvis

*Attachment points of
the deep muscles*

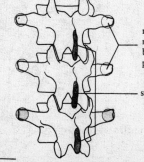

note that the tendons of
most of the muscles in the
back are attached to the bony
processes of the vertebrae

spine

Three vertebrae superimposed

(*iii*)   *The abdominal muscles*

You will see from the following diagrams that it is the oblique muscles of the abdomen which allow you to bend and rotate your upper body and help it to bend forward.

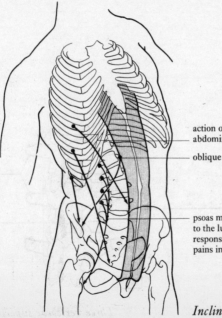

action of the oblique
abdominal muscles

oblique muscle

psoas muscle, attached
to the lumbar vertebrae,
responsible for certain
pains in the lumbar region

Inclination of the trunk to the right side

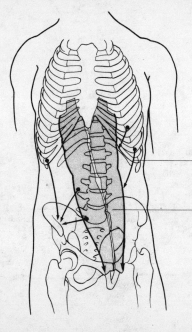

action of the oblique
muscles

rectus abdominus
muscle

the action of the
rectus abdominus
muscle predominates

the rectus abdominus
to the front, the
oblique muscles to
the rear

Rotation of the trunk

Flexion of the trunk to the front

8 The ligaments of the spinal column

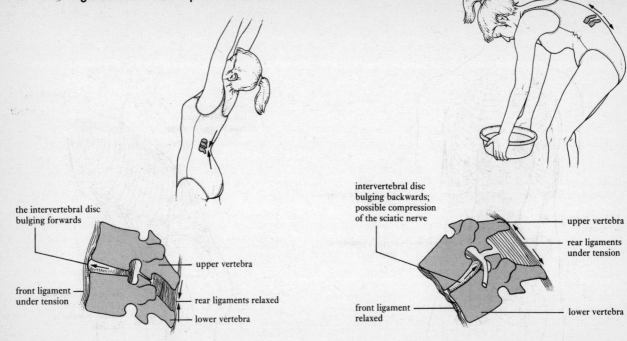

the intervertebral disc
bulging forwards

front ligament
under tension

upper vertebra

rear ligaments relaxed

lower vertebra

Approximation of vertebrae posteriorly

intervertebral disc
bulging backwards;
possible compression
of the sciatic nerve

front ligament
relaxed

upper vertebra

rear ligaments
under tension

lower vertebra

Separation of vertebrae posteriorly

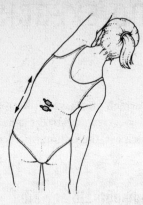

9 The nervous system

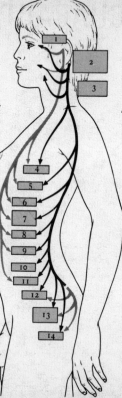

Parasympathetic system

Sympathetic system

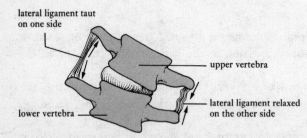

lateral ligament taut on one side

upper vertebra

lower vertebra

lateral ligament relaxed on the other side

Lateral separation

1 eye
2 lacrymal and salivary glands
3 head capillaries
4 lung
5 heart
6 stomach
7 liver and gall-bladder
8 pancreas
9 kidney
10 suprarenals
11 intestines
12 bladder
13 genital organs
14 rectum

THE CHARACTERISTICS OF WA-DO EXERCISES

Remember, Wa-Do exercises are the ones which you have all been searching for *instinctively*. They are *your exercises*. They correspond to those needs of the body which we should satisfy if we are to achieve the optimum efficiency and well-being that we are looking for.

1 Anywhere, any time, in a few moments, in any kind of clothing

Wa-Do exercises may be practised *anywhere*: in bed, at our place of work, in the car, sitting in a train or aeroplane, in the bath, on the grass, or in the gym . . .

Any time: We don't need any special apparatus. We can practise the exercises according to which position suits us at the time: sitting, standing, lying down, or on all fours.

In a few moments: 10 seconds to 1 minute are enough to find relief. We can repeat the exercises as many times a day as we like, without any waste of time, and some exercises can even be performed while we are getting on with everyday business – answering the telephone, watching the television or writing, for example.

In any kind of clothing: there is no need to get dressed up to do Wa-Do exercises. Whatever clothes you have on will be fine; just be sure to loosen your shirt collar or belt a little so that you can breathe more comfortably.

The following advice will enable you to exercise safely with the best results.

2   The essential principle of pleasant sensitivity

Pain makes us tense, and this impairs good circulation to the affected area. If the nerve cells are not properly supplied with blood and nutrients, particularly oxygen, this prolongs the painful condition and the poor functioning of the organs they control. By improving the circulation to the nerve cells we can break the vicious circle of pain and discomfort.

When you hurt yourself, you instinctively put your hand on the painful place to get relief. When you feel stiff in the joints, you instinctively move them to make them feel better.

WE ALL KNOW, INSTINCTIVELY, THAT PARTICULAR STATE OF SENSI-TIVENESS OR PLEASURABLE PAIN THAT SOOTHES US.

Each exercise is therefore performed:
- *gently:* without forcing and without any abrupt or jerky movement

● *in comfort:* first of all find a suitable position for the exercise – one that causes you the least pain, and may even bring relief or make you feel good

● *with caution:* perform the exercise slowly at first, and gradually find out the most suitable pace for you

● *sensitively:* follow and consciously feel the movement all the time you are performing it

● *with repetition:* the same exercise should be repeated 10 times (less when there is pain), then start again in 2 or 3 series of 10; the duration of each exercise varies between 1 and 5 seconds on average

● *symmetrically:* most of the exercises should be performed 10 times on one side (in 2 or 3 series), then repeated on the other side; always begin with the less sensitive side.

3 Using the weight of your body

Using the weight of your body has a number of advantages:

● *simplicity:* the weight of the whole body or part of it, without using any other equipment, allows you to get the movement under way and maintain it

● *ease:* there is no need to force the movement; you should feel quite comfortable performing it

● *direct awareness of your body:* any tension, contraction or 'knotted' feeling will be immediately detectable, and, according to your physical condition at the time, can increase the feeling of heaviness which indicates that more exercise is needed.

4   Acquiring automatic movement through the elasticity of body tissues

All the living tissues of the body have one essential quality: elasticity (old age and death harden them). In the same way that a rubber band yields to force, the tissues can stretch to a certain point. But, unlike the rubber band, the living structure of our body, with appropriate training, can acquire a greater degree of elasticity. It's a matter of finding the right *training rhythm*. It's a combination of the pleasurable feeling of sensitivity and the sensation of well-being that imparts it.

By repeating an exercise 10 times or so, the elasticity of the tissues produces an *automatic movement* on demand, so to speak. It comes about spontaneously, with very little fatigue and with the advantage that you exercise only minimum voluntary control.

IF YOU FEEL ANY KIND OF DISCOMFORT, PAIN OR FATIGUE WHEN PERFORMING AN EXERCISE, YOU MUST SLOW DOWN, REDUCE MOVEMENT, OR MOVE INTO A MORE COMFORTABLE POSITION.

5   The extent and speed of the movements

It is the elasticity of the tissues or organs mobilized in any particular exercise which determine the size and speed of the movement involved. You must take care to perform the exercise slowly at first, without any jerkiness and with a limited range of movement. As soon as there is some improvement in your condition the range of movement can be increased, but you should still go slowly.

Once the exercise can be performed smoothly and harmoniously, you can increase the speed naturally.

The exercises should always be performed in a supple, relaxed manner, almost without thinking about them.

6   Breathing follows movement, while adapting to it

Always keep your mouth half open to inhale and exhale, breathing through your mouth and nose at the same time, except where otherwise indicated.

As a general rule, instinct will guide us:

●   to exhale when the body folds over and the limbs come together
●   to inhale when the body unfolds and the limbs move apart.

Each exercise is performed (except where otherwise indicated) during one complete inhalation–exhalation cycle, as will be clearly explained in the text.

7   Relief followed by strengthening

All the everyday cases of pain or discomfort are tackled in two parts:
- exercises to relieve the condition
- exercises to strengthen.

Chapters which do not follow this pattern include those on obesity and underweight, pain in the joints and muscles due to premature ageing, and various problems and pains associated with long periods of study.

Before beginning the second part of each chapter (strengthening exercises), it is recommended that you repeat the movements of the first part (exercises for relief) to ensure the best results.

BASIC EXERCISES

A gentle, rocking kind of movement is essential to all Wa-Do exercises. Start the initial impulse and let it run like a wave throughout your whole body. All the exercises should be performed in a completely relaxed, automatic manner, employing the minimum effort.

1   To stretch the tendons and loosen up the joints

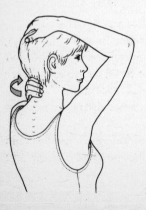

Put your body into the exact position shown in the illustration and use the reduced elasticity of the tendons and ligaments. *The exercise is performed within a very limited circle of movement, practically without any effort.* Your breathing should be shallow.

Example:
Turn your head to the right and put your right hand on the top of your head, with your right arm relaxed. Place your left hand around the top part of the back of your neck, and let your first three fingers curl around the protruding portion of the vertebral column.

- as you lower your left elbow, your head will turn just a little bit more to the right; exhale
- as you lift your left elbow slightly, your head will turn just a little bit more to the left; inhale.

The head movements are quite small.

2   To relax the muscles

Adopting a neutral position (see p. 50), use the ability of the muscle fibres to lengthen and shorten: *the movement should be large and ample in scope.* Breathing should be heavier and deeper than in the previous exercise.

Example (almost identical to the previous one but involving a different action):
Put your head in neutral position (nose along the central line of your body), and your right hand on the top of your head with your arm relaxed; your left hand is placed around the top part of the back of your neck, and the first three fingers curl around the protruding portion of your vertebral column.

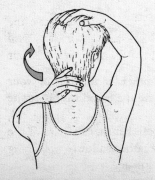

- as you lower your left elbow, turn your head in a large circular movement towards the right; exhale during the movement
- as you raise your left elbow to its original position, your head should return to the neutral position with a large circular movement to the left; inhale during the movement.

In this exercise your head movements should be large.

3 To release nervous pressure and improve the circulation

To release nervous pressure it helps to improve the circulation serving the nervous pathways. It all comes down to action affecting the blood supply. We use an action which is like pumping the blood: *the exercise entails a phase of compression followed by an interval of maintained pressure, then a phase of relaxing pressure.*

Note that pressure is applied progressively to reach a particular feeling of 'pleasurable sensitivity or pain'. Never go beyond a point where the pain becomes acute or unpleasant.

Exhale while releasing the pressure.

Breathe shallowly during the interval of maintained pressure.

Inhale as you release the pressure.

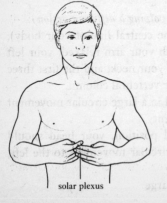

solar plexus

Example:

Place the fingers of one hand over those of the other at the top of your abdomen under the point of the sternum, and increase the blood supply to the solar plexus.

● apply progressive pressure with the fingers of both hands; exhale
● maintain the pressure for a few moments and breathe shallowly
● gradually release the pressure on the abdomen; inhale

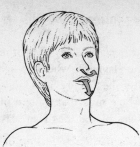

4 To improve respiration

There are three types of respiration:

A *Superficial spontaneous respiration*

We often stop breathing without realizing it: we block the simplest form of respiration that is so vital to life. To help our respiration to function more freely, we must keep our mouth partly open to allow the air to enter it.

B *Complete thoracic respiration*

This calls upon all the muscular structures and activates the rib cage. For convenience we can divide it into four stages (during one complete inhalation of breath):

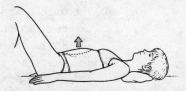

(i) *abdominal breathing:* in expanding the lower region of the lungs, the diaphragm muscle contracts and pushes down the abdomen, which expands in turn

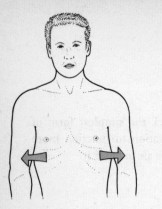

(ii) *medium thoracic respiration:* this is attained by enlarging the rib cage by means of the intercostal and pectoral muscles

(iii) *high clavicular respiration:* for this we use our neck muscles to lift the uppermost part of the thorax, and in particular the clavicles; when we are short of air, we can perform this kind of breathing after the two previous kinds

(iv) *complete respiration:* this calls into play the whole muscular system of the body to effect a complete stretching; the muscles of the toes also play their part in this exercise (see illustration on p. 49).

C *Respiration of the pulmonary apparatus*

● the pelvis and the diaphragm are strongly activated during deep inhalation and exhalation

● the trachea, and the bronchioles, which are part of it, benefit from the action of prolonged inhalation and exhalation; to achieve this we push our lips forwards while breathing through them

● the pulmonary alveolar sacs, which are directly in contact with the blood vessels, can also be brought into play in a voluntary fashion. After forced inhalation, hold your breath in. Push the trapped air to the top of your lungs to dilate the upper alveolar sacs; then push the trapped air down to the bottom of your lungs to dilate the lower alveolar sacs.

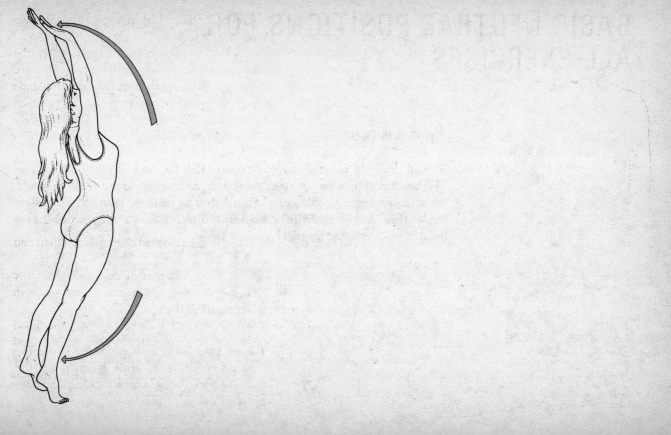

BASIC NEUTRAL POSITIONS FOR ALL EXERCISES

Lying positions

For all the lying positions we must ensure that the back of the neck (not just the head) is supported, to avoid tension or contraction in the neck. It would be a good thing if people made this a habit, so that, for example, the pillow under their ears or under their head in bed did not make their neck act as a kind of bridge during the night.

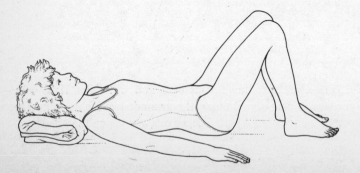

Lie on your back, with a cushion under the back of your neck, arms lying along the sides of your body, knees together and feet apart.

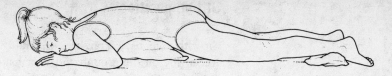

Lie on your stomach, with a cushion under your abdomen and your ankles. Turn your head to the side where one arm is folded upwards; stretch the other arm comfortably along the opposite side of your body.

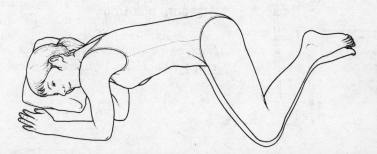

Lie on one side, with a cushion under your neck and with your right arm folded under your neck or stretched along the ground; bend your left arm with your hand on the ground; bend your legs, resting one leg on the other.

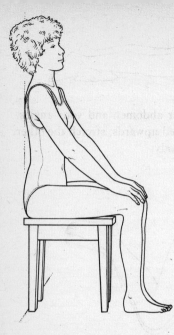

Sitting position

Sit with your back straight – preferably leaning against something; place your feet firmly on the ground and your hands on your thighs. Put your head in a neutral position, looking straight ahead; and relax your shoulders.

All-fours position

Stretch your arms, to keep your back flat; raise your head and look straight ahead.

Standing position

Leaning against a wall allows a gradual progression of movement with the minimum of fatigue. Press your trunk nice and straight against the wall, pushing out the hollow at the bottom of your back. Stretch your legs, with your feet resting on the ground, with the width of your shoulders between them, about 2 inches from the wall.

PRACTICE PROGRAMME

1   The universal nature of Wa-Do exercises

By strengthening all our organic functions and developing our personal vitality, Wa-Do exercises help restore calm, self-control, receptiveness and energy, no matter what our actual physical condition or state of mind might be. When our vital energy is properly channelled it becomes clear that:

● a sick person is just a well person who is unaware of his true self (except in extreme cases)
● every fit person should be responsible for maintaining his basic physical and mental functions in order to remain healthy
● developing our individual faculties is a source of pleasure.

2   The criteria of their effectiveness

Wa-Do exercises are simple, precise, clear and reliable. They require only *a sensitive awareness* of the movements being performed. The effectiveness of

the exercises and the improvement they produce are always indicated by:
- relief from the upset, tiredness or pain
- local or regional disappearance of the feeling of fatigue
- greater ease of movement
- local or regional appearance of a feeling of vigour and gentle warmth, produced by an improved blood supply.

These signs can appear almost instantly – within only 10 seconds of a series of movements. We can then pass on to a more advanced stage of exercise.

3   The order of body positions

This is very important: results will be *more rapid* if exercises are followed in the correct order.

For the sake of clarity let us make a comparison. A baby depends instinctively on its increase in vitality and on the precision of its nervous system to pass successively from a lying to a sitting position, then to all-fours, and finally to standing up. The development of its body operates progressively, without any waste of energy or needless fatigue, towards maximum efficiency. Let's protect our nervous system by following a similar cycle of development:
- a lying down position
- a sitting position
- a squatting or all-fours position
- a standing position.

Most of the time, away from home, only the sitting and standing positions are easy to perform. However, *in cases of extreme pain, the standing position should be avoided*, and for this reason *the sitting position will be the most common*. Once back home, or as soon as possible, follow the order indicated, starting with the lying position. In this way you will lay the most solid foundations for rapid and lasting results.

4 Rest between the series of movements

It is beneficial to rest for a while between each series of movements. The length of this rest period depends on how tired you feel: generally speaking a few seconds are enough, but you may need 1–2 minutes.

5 Rhythm and duration of exercises

(*i*) *For those with problems*
If you begin to experience pain or a relatively minor problem, practise a series of 10 movements of 1–5 seconds' duration, in other words 10 seconds to 1 minute in all. This should ease the problem. Repeat as necessary.

In cases of recent or persistent pain you should practise:
● a series of 10 movements to improve the local circulation

- a series of 10 movements to improve the circulation to the nervous system
- a series of 10 movements to improve your respiration.

Punctuate each series with a pause of a few seconds (5–10), i.e. 1–3 minutes pause altogether.

For symptoms that have been experienced over a long time, only repetition of the exercises will bring about a progressive improvement and long-lasting results:

- repeat one series of exercises several times a day, no matter where you are; in all, several sessions of between 10 seconds and 1 minute each
- if you set aside 5–10 minutes each morning to perform the exercises, you will be rewarded with good health.

(*ii*) *For those in good health and for sporting enthusiasts*

This method uses strengthening exercises that make the body feel more comfortable; it produces maximum recovery, and can even improve the performance of athletes engaged in competition. Various kinds of pain in the back, neck and shoulders, digestive problems and nervous disorders are very common in this group of people. Students, young or old (see p. 368), are advised to make their bodies as fit as possible for prolonged study. Everybody, irrespective of age, should choose suitable exercises to prevent the onset of bothersome aches and pains and to consolidate their general health. For preventative action and to develop the health generally, a session of 10–20 minutes every 2 days seems the best pattern to adopt.

6 Liquid intake

Most of us have got into the bad habit of not drinking enough liquid, and it is strongly recommended that you drink one or more glasses of water after exercising for more than 15 minutes. If you drink fruit or vegetable juices, you are taking in vitamins as well.

7 Gentle, systematic training of the body is the basis for good health

The majority of occupations and professions do not call for physical effort of an intense or brief nature. More often than not, our muscles have to maintain fixed postures or perform repetitive movements for many hours a day. Only gentle, systematic training can be of physiological benefit. It does not tire the body, it develops the necessary physiological and metabolic reflexes, it relieves aches and pains, and it replenishes energy – without producing the exhaustion or crippling stiffness that follow intensive physical exercise.

THE OBJECTIVE IS A DEEP AND LASTING FEELING OF WELL–BEING THROUGHOUT THE WHOLE BODY, OF CALM ENERGY, OF BEING COMPLETELY RELAXED.

In cases of persistent health problems, or if they worsen, or in any case of doubt, it is, of course, recommended that you consult your doctor.

WA-DO:
THE WAY TO FEELING GOOD

The exercises shown in this section of the book are only a tiny proportion of those that our body is capable of performing, and have been chosen for their simplicity. I am sure you will discover a multitude of variations in rhythm, breadth of movement and combination: make these your own exercises.

It's your turn now.

And don't forget: relax. *Never force it*.

●   for all the exercises: keep your mouth open

➡   a tinted arrow indicates a movement

→   a black arrow indicates pressure exerted

HEADACHE

Migraine

This is a universal complaint. When it's coming on, you have an empty feeling in your head, bright flashes in front of your eyes, and nausea. Then the storm breaks: an intense pain strikes on one side of your skull, at the front of the temple. You may start vomiting. You can't bear noise or light. All physical or mental effort seems impossible. To tell the truth, you are often expecting it: you shouldn't have had that chocolate or that wine . . . you shouldn't have spent so long over those figures . . . or maybe it's the new moon . . .

/ *Exercises for relief*

1 To calm the digestion

Directly over the region of the stomach, liver and gall-bladder, at the solar plexus, is the junction of the nerves which control them. In the following

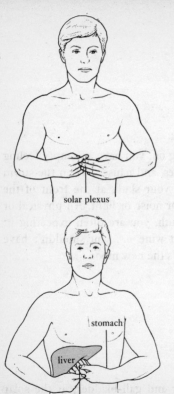

solar plexus

stomach

liver

gall-bladder

exercise you improve the digestion, the elimination of toxins, and the decongestion of the liver, to which the venous blood of the intestines passes before returning to the heart.

Lean your body slightly forward and place the fingers of one hand over those of the other at the top of your abdomen.
- steadily increase the pressure; exhale
- maintain the pressure; breathe shallowly
- steadily decrease the pressure; inhale
- repeat the exercise 10 times.

Sitting down with your body leaning slightly forwards, curl your fingers round under your right ribs (liver, gall-bladder).
- gradually increase the pressure, penetrating beneath the ribs; exhale
- maintain the pressure and breathe shallowly, then gradually release pressure, drawing your fingers out; inhale
- repeat the exercise 10 times
- do the same under your left ribs (stomach).

2   To improve respiration

This exercise will increase the flow of oxygen-rich blood to your head and face.

Adopt one of the positions described on p. 55, and put your hands over your solar plexus.
● contract your throat and breathe in with little gulps
● repeat the exercises 10 times.

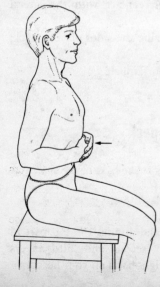

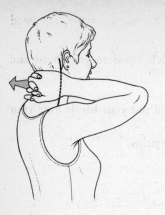

3   To improve the circulation of the blood to the head

This exercise applies gentle pressure, on and off, to the pathways of the autonomic nerves passing over the sides of your neck which act upon the circulation to the brain.

Place your hands, with fingers interlocked, over the nape of your neck and relax your arms with the fleshy part of the palms in contact with the lateral muscles.

- bring your palms and elbows together, squeezing the sides of your neck; exhale
- move your elbows apart and take the pressure off; inhale
- repeat the exercise 10 times.

4 To relax and loosen up the back of the neck

These exercises operate in particular on the muscles at the base of the skull.

To relax the tendons

Turn your head to the right and curl your left hand around the top part of your neck; with your arm relaxed, hook the first, second and third fingers round the ridge of the vertebral column. Put your right hand on your head.

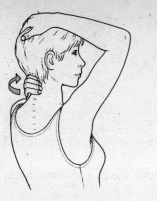

- lower your left elbow, stretch the back of your neck and make your head turn a little more; exhale
- raise your elbow, letting the head turn back; inhale
- after a series of 10 movements, reverse the procedure for the other side.

To loosen up the muscles

Put your head in a neutral position, with your hands in the same position as in the previous exercise.
- turn your head and neck to the right; exhale
- let the head return; inhale
- after a series of 10 movements, reverse the procedure for the other side.

5 Menstrual headaches, see *Premenstrual syndrome*, p. 312.

II *Strengthening exercises*

1 The digestion

This is an exercise to improve the blood supply to the pathways of the autonomic nerves in the middle of the neck controlling the digestion.

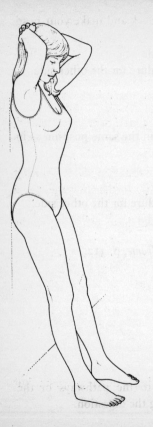

Sit down and put your left hand flat between your back and the back of your chair.
● let yourself go backwards, or lean more strongly against the back of the seat; inhale
● maintain the pressure; breathe shallowly
● relax the pressure by gently leaning forwards; exhale; treat the groups of muscles in the middle of the back in the same way
● after a series of 10 movements, reverse the procedure for the other side.

VARIATION: Use your fist for greater pressure.

autonomic nervous pathways

2   Respiration

Exaggerating the movements of your diaphragm helps to get rid of the sensation of having a lump 'in the pit of your stomach'.

Place your hands a little behind the crown of your head.
● inhale, pulling your chin back into your chest and contracting your neck
● hold your breath for a few moments
● relax the contraction in your neck; exhale
● repeat the exercise 10 times.

3 Circulation

This exercise applies pressure, on and off, to the nervous pathways controlling the blood supply to your brain, while moving your head to the left and the right.

Place your hands over the nape of your neck with your fingers interlocked; relax your arms, the fleshy part of your palms in contact with the lateral muscles of the neck.

- take your left elbow downwards and to the right, squeezing with your left hand; exhale; the right elbow will rise in response to the movement and your head will turn to the right
- bring your left elbow to its starting position, your head returning to the front; release the pressure; inhale
- after a series of 10 movements, reverse the procedure for the other side.

4 To relax and loosen up the neck

Relaxing

This uses the same movements as described in Exercises 3 and 4 on p. 64, but applied to the top of your neck.

autonomic nervous
pathway

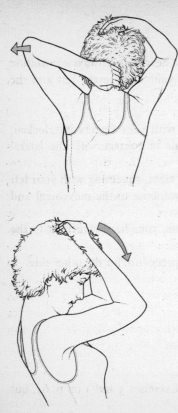

Loosening up

Curl your left hand round the right side of your neck; with your right hand placed on the top of your head.
● incline your head to the right, then, when it has gone as far as it can, gently pull it a little further with your left hand; exhale
● release the pressure; inhale
● after a series of 10 movements, reverse the procedure for the other side.

Place your hands on the top of your head and draw in your chin.
● draw your chin in more by pressing down on your head with both hands; exhale
● relax the pressure; inhale
● repeat the procedure 10 times.

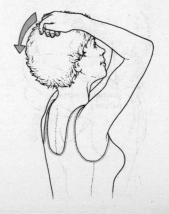

Put your hands on the top of your head and then throw your head back.
● accentuate the movement of your head by pressing it with both hands; inhale
● let your head come back; exhale
● repeat the procedure 10 times.

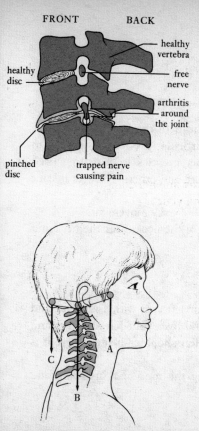

healthy vertebra

free nerve

arthritis around the joint

healthy disc

pinched disc

trapped nerve causing pain

FRONT   BACK

A

B

C

Cervical spondylosis

Once past the age of 40 you could be afflicted by this physiological ailment. You may go a long time without suffering any symptoms, then suddenly certain ordinary movements (for example a simple action like reversing the car) can unleash pains in your neck which may extend upwards to your head or outwards to your shoulders.

Because it is strategically placed within the mechanism of the brain's circulation, this type of arthritis can produce a whole range of quite disagreeable symptoms: frequent headaches, feelings of unsteadiness and dizziness, buzzing in the ears, or a sudden giving way of the legs when you bend your neck backwards. If the condition affects the nerves of your arms, you will have pain that radiates from your neck to your hand, or pins and needles in your fingers (cervico-brachial neuralgia). And because of the muscular relationship between the back of your neck and the top of your back, you may feel sharp stabbing pains in this area, leading you to suspect a heart problem.

Cervical spondylosis is caused by the head's weight (A) straining forwards off the vertebral axis (B), causing a permanent contraction of the neck muscles (C) which squeezes the cervical vertebrae on top of one another. It just shows that even though a human being is well constructed, he's not quite perfect!

Left: Leverage system of the head

/ *Exercises for relief*

1   To relax and loosen up

The superficial muscles that stretch from the head to the back, for example the trapezius and the levator scapulae, are particularly effective, thanks to their length of leverage; they prevent the deeper muscles from getting tired needlessly. Stretching and relaxing them – before any others – brings instant relief.

● one hand will support and absorb any possible jerky movements
● note that the cervical vertebrae at the base of the neck, near the back and less mobile, are the ones mostly affected.

To relax the tendons

Put your head in the neutral position. Bend your left arm with your left hand pressed against your side; stretch your right hand over your left shoulder and curl your fingers round the bony ridge of your left shoulder–blade, where it is attached to the trapezius.

● slightly lower your right elbow, stretching the muscular insertion, and making your head turn a little; exhale
● bring your elbow upwards; inhale
● repeat the procedure 10 times

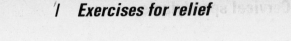

lower attachment
of levator scapulae

bony ridge of
shoulderblade

lower attachment
of trapezius

attachment of
deep muscles

- proceed all along the bony ridge, and also on the inner corner of your shoulder-blade, where another muscle is attached and is generally in a state of contraction: the levator anguli scapulae
- finish in the area between your shoulder-blade and your spine, to reach the deep muscles
- repeat the procedure on the other side, reversing the position of your hands.

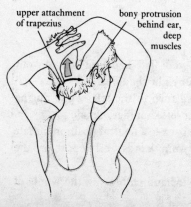

upper attachment of trapezius

bony protrusion behind ear, deep muscles

Put your head in the neutral position and interlock your fingers on the top of your skull. Put the thumb of your left hand in the bony depression at the base of your skull, where the trapezius and other muscles are attached.

- apply pressure with the help of your left thumb in the depression and bend your neck to the right to make your scalp and the muscular insertion slide over the surface of the bone; exhale, and feel the skin sliding over the surface of your skull
- bring your elbow back upwards; inhale
- repeat the procedure 10 times
- do the same thing all along the depression and stop at the bony protrusion behind your ear, where other muscles are inserted
- repeat on the other side, reversing the position of your hands.

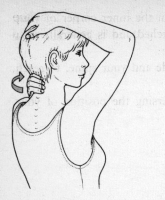

Turn your head to the right, and with your left hand at the base of your neck hook your first three fingers round the lower cervical vertebrae; place your other hand palm downwards on your head.

● lower your left elbow, bringing it down slightly to the right, stretching the insertions of the tendons and making your head turn slightly; inhale
● raise your elbow, relaxing your head and bringing it back to its normal position; exhale
● after a series of 10 movements, reverse the position of your hands and repeat on the other side.

To relax the muscles

Put your head in the neutral position. Place your left hand on top of your skull, curl your right hand round the top of your right shoulder.

● lower your right elbow to make your head turn to the left, while raising your chin so as not to knock it against your left shoulder; exhale
● raise your right elbow, bringing your head back to a neutral position; inhale
● after a series of 10 movements, reverse your hands and repeat on the other side
● do the same exercise with the palm of your hand embracing the whole of the back of your neck.

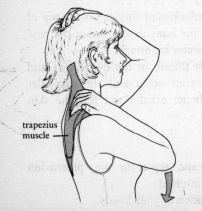

trapezius
muscle

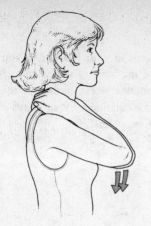

Put your head in the neutral position, with both hands curling round the top of your back on either side of your neck, between your shoulder-blades and your spine.

- lower both elbows at the same time, keeping your head straight; exhale, and feel the trapezius and the deep muscles stretching
- bring your elbows back up; inhale
- repeat the movement 10 times.

2 To improve breathing

It is good to breathe in a way that makes the lower part of the neck work. We can do this by accentuating the movement of the upper chest.

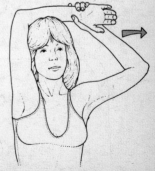

Put both your arms above your head and let your left hand take hold of your right wrist; turn your head slightly to the left, so that it rests in the angle of your right elbow.

- with your left hand draw your right wrist to the left while breathing in; inhale
- relax; exhale
- after a series of 10 movements, reverse hands and repeat on the other side; note that the front muscles of the neck assist breathing in the upper chest.

3   To improve circulation

Depending on whether you have circulation problems in your head or in your arms, work on either the top or the bottom part of the back of your neck. By applying gentle pressure, on and off, to the autonomic nerve pathways that travel over the sides of your neck, you act on the circulation to your brain or on your arm circulation and its nerves (see *Circulation*, p. 67).

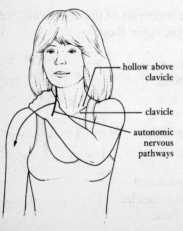

hollow above clavicle

clavicle

autonomic nervous pathways

When the problems are mainly in your head
Work on the top of your neck (see *Migraine*, p. 67–8).

When the problems are in your arms
Stretch your left hand over your right shoulder.
● press on the hollow above your clavicle against the shoulder muscle; exhale
● maintain the pressure and breathe shallowly
● relax the pressure; inhale
● after a series of 10 movements, reverse hands and repeat on the other side.

// *Strengthening exercises*

1 To relax and loosen up

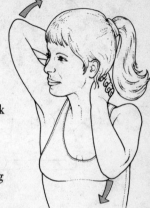

Relaxing

With both hands, one on top of the other, cover the back of your neck; turn your head to the right and raise your chin, lower your left elbow, and raise your right one.
- slightly accentuate the rotational movement by raising your right elbow a little higher and lowering your left one; inhale
- relax the tension; exhale
- repeat the procedure 10 times
- apply the same movements over the length of your neck
- reverse the movements for the other side.

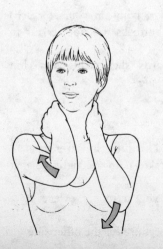

Loosening up

Position your hands as in the previous exercise. This time, however, put your head in the neutral position, your hands round the back of your neck, and your elbows in front of your chest.
- lower your left elbow and raise your right one, with your chin rising towards the right; inhale

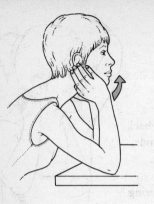

- return to the central position, with both elbows at the same height in front of your chest; exhale
- repeat the movement 10 times
- apply the same treatment over the length of your neck
- reverse the procedure for the other side.

To improve flexibility of the joints

Lean with your elbows on a table (or on the floor, lying on your stomach) and put your palms under your chin; keep your buttocks well to the rear to stretch your neck.

- with chin raised and your head bent backwards, slightly lift your chin upwards by pushing it up with your hands; exhale
- stop pushing; inhale
- repeat the operation 10 times.

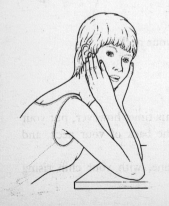

Use the same position as in the previous exercise. This time, however, instead of having your chin to the front, your left hand takes it to the right, so that your face is turned towards the right and upward.

- push your chin slightly towards the right with your left hand; exhale
- stop pushing; inhale
- after a series of 10 movements, reverse the procedure for the other side.

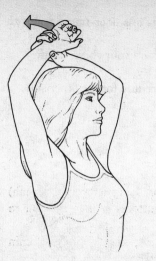

2   To improve breathing

These exercises work on the deep muscles at the top of the back, reducing as much as possible the weight exerted by the arms and the head.

With both arms above your head, take hold of your right wrist with your left arm, with your head slightly turned to the left.
● with your left hand draw your right wrist backwards; inhale
● relax; exhale
● after a series of 10 movements, reverse the procedure for the other side.

Lie down on a bed, with the back of your neck supported by a pillow and the top of your neck resting on the corner of the bed or on one of its side edges. Let your arms hang relaxed off the bed, and keep your legs bent.
● let your arms fall back a little more; inhale
● let them spring up again; exhale
● repeat the exercise 10 times.

VARIATION: Do the same exercise holding a weight of 1 or 2 kilos in your hands to accentuate the movement.

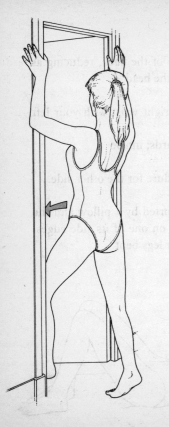

Stand up, placing your forearms against the uprights of a door-frame and with one foot in front of the other.

- slightly bend your front leg – this will help expand your chest; inhale
- straighten up again while stretching your front leg
- after a series of 10 movements, reverse the procedure for the other side.

3   To improve circulation

This exercise applies pressure on and off to the group of muscles at the back of your neck.

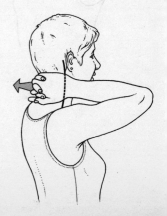

Place your hands over the back of your neck with fingers interlocked and arms relaxed.

- lift the skin and the muscles of the back of your neck by drawing the palms of your hands together; exhale
- relax; inhale
- repeat the exercise 10 times.

Tension in the back of the neck and in the shoulders

Working in fixed postures, holding our arms in the same position for a long time, or making repetitive movements, can often lead to intolerable pain at the back of our neck and in our shoulders. This can produce a sensation of heaviness, with burning or 'gnawing' feelings in the affected area, and the pain is often accompanied by a heavy feeling at the back of the head. These feelings can be intensely irritating, sapping us physically and lowering our morale. Typists, hairdressers, dentists, people who concentrate on high precision work, and many others, know these problems only too well and come to dread them.

/ *Exercises for relief*

1   To improve respiration

Any kind of hard work requires a good supply of oxygen to the muscles. Practise breathing exercises while reducing as much as possible the weight exerted by your arms and head.

See *Cervical spondylosis*, pp. 73, 77.

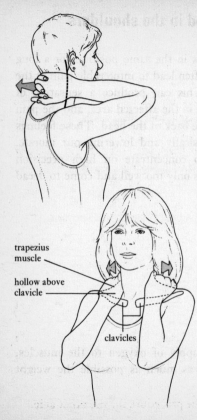

trapezius
muscle

hollow above
clavicle

clavicles

2 To improve circulation

These exercises apply pressure on and off to the group of muscles serving the back of your neck and your shoulders.

Place your hands over the back of your neck with your fingers interlocked and your arms relaxed.

● squeeze the muscles of the back of your neck by drawing the palms of your hands together; exhale
● maintain the pressure; breathe shallowly
● release the pressure; inhale
● repeat the exercise 10 times.

Place the palm of each hand over the trapezius muscle at the top of your shoulders.

● apply pressure on the trapezius on each side of the depression above the clavicle; exhale
● release the pressure; inhale
● repeat the exercise 10 times.

VARIATION: With your right arm relaxed, put your right hand around the left trapezius muscle.

● after a series of 10 movements, reverse the procedure for the other side.

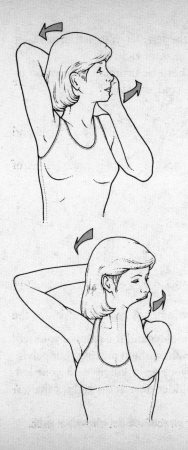

// *Strengthening exercises*

To relax

Turning your head to the left, raise your chin to the most comfortable position; put your left hand under your chin, and your right hand on your left temple.
- slightly exaggerate the movement of your head, with the hand under your chin pushing to the left and the right hand bringing your temple round to the right; exhale
- relax; inhale
- after a series of 10 movements, reverse the procedure for the other side.

Turn your head to the left, lower your chin and stretch the back of your neck in a comfortable position; put your left hand under your chin, with your right hand on your left temple.
- slightly accentuate the movement of your head, the hand under your chin pressing to the left and your right hand bringing your temple round to the right; exhale
- release the pressure; inhale
- after a series of 10 movements, reverse the procedure for the other side.

From a neutral position, incline your head to the left; let your left arm reach round your head so that your left hand can rest on your right ear.
- slightly accentuate the movement of your head by bringing it down on to your left shoulder with the aid of your left hand; exhale
- release the pressure; inhale
- after a series of 10 movements, reverse the procedure for the other side.

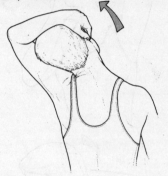

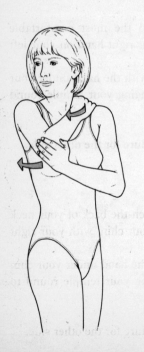

Place the palm of your right hand on your left shoulder and the palm of your left hand on your right elbow; turn your trunk to the right without moving your pelvis.
- accentuate the movement by pushing on your right elbow with your left hand. This makes the whole of the left shoulder turn to the right; exhale
- release the pressure; inhale
- after a series of 10 movements, reverse the procedure for the other side.

2 To loosen up

Put your arms behind your back; take hold of your left wrist with your right hand and lean your head slightly backwards.
- bring your shoulder-blades together by pulling against your left wrist with your right hand, and let your head tilt back more; inhale
- release the traction; exhale
- after a series of 10 movements, reverse the procedure for the other side.

Sit down and put your left hand on the seat of your chair, with your right hand resting on the inner part of your right thigh; turn your trunk to the left, raising your chin.
- push on your thigh with your right hand, supporting yourself on it to increase the momentum of your trunk towards the left. This will bring your head towards your right shoulder and loosen up the muscles at the top of your back; exhale
- stop pushing and allow your head, shoulders and trunk to return to their original position; inhale
- after a series of 10 movements, repeat the procedure for the other side.

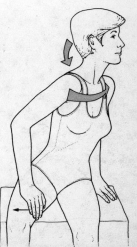

Place your hands palm downwards on the edge of a desk; lean forward and bend your elbows so that you feel your shoulder-blades coming together.
● push down on your hands to raise your chest; exhale
● let your chest drop back on to the desk – this contracts the muscles of your back; inhale
● repeat the exercise 10 times.

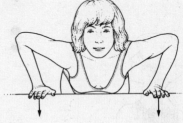

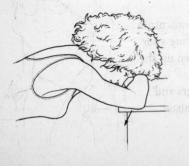

With your elbows bent on the edge of the desk, and your hands resting one on top of the other, place your forehead on your hands, sitting far enough back in the chair to have your back stretched.
● push backwards and down on your elbows without disturbing your head – this loosens up the muscles in your back; exhale
● relax; inhale, and feel your muscles loosening
● repeat the exercise 10 times.

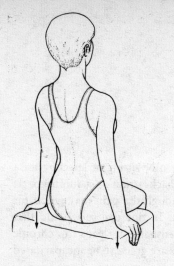

Sit down and place your hands on each side of your buttocks.
- push on your hands and lower your shoulders, as though to grow taller – this will contract the group of dorsal muscles; inhale
- relax; exhale; feel your muscles loosen
- repeat the exercise 10 times.

3 To improve respiration

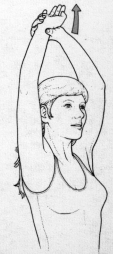

Bend your arms behind your head, and take hold of your right wrist with your left hand.
- push upwards with both hands to stretch your arms, keeping them as far as possible behind your head – this will bring your head backwards slightly; inhale
- let your hands and arms return to the starting position behind your head; exhale
- repeat the exercise 10 times.

BACK PROBLEMS

Pains in the lumbar area

After lifting a heavy object, or getting up quickly after sitting or kneeling for a long time, we may suddenly be seized with 'back strain', or lumbago. It usually puts us out of action for a few days, although the pain may go on for weeks, well after our return to normal activities. In due course we find that the problem occurs again and again, and eventually it leads to chronic lumbago. When this happens we don't know if we are going to be incapacitated from one day to the next.

Sometimes the situation is even more serious. Following some difficult work that we are not used to, or perhaps a long car journey, an intense, searing pain shoots through our back. The slightest movement is agony, and the pain can sometimes reach our buttocks or even our feet. This is an attack of sciatica, for which the only treatment is a few weeks' lying down. Unfortunately, after such an incident, there is always the fear of a recurrence.

In both the above cases the pain is due to the crushing of an intervertebral disc and the resulting pressure on the nerves.

We may also suffer from less severe and more familiar discomforts: tension around the lumbar region accompanying intestinal spasms or flatulence, that feeling of being 'completely full up' when we are depressed; and with women, a heaviness in the lower back around the time of their period. But most of us just put up with it – we get used to it.

It is absolutely essential to rest completely during such an attack, of course. But once the pain has subsided, we must start strengthening this fragile part of our body. As two-legged creatures, we must not forget that our back has to carry a large proportion of our weight.

Obesity, bad posture and weakness in the muscles and ligaments of the back, abdomen, legs and feet predispose us to back problems. During the last few decades back trouble has become the 'complaint of our time'; but isn't it more the 'complaint of our legs' or the 'complaint of our abdomen'? Our balance relies, in fact, on the strength and good co-ordination of our legs. They have played an essential role, since our infancy, in the way we stand up, walk, jump, run or climb. The large gluteal muscle is a pillar in our body architecture that supports the whole of our upper body. What is more, it has the distinction of being the body's largest and most powerful muscle. When ill-used and stiffened by sedentary life, it can no longer guarantee to perform its proper function and surrenders its role to other muscles, which are poor substitutes. The common contractions and pains which people experience in their lower backs are the result.

A tree spreads with solid roots beneath it. It's the same with our body: its roots are our legs. Let's take care of them for our back's sake.

Chronic abdominal trouble tends to make us stoop, and can easily lead to pain in the lower back. So keep a watchful eye on the healthy function of your abdominal organs.

When our leg muscles – and in particular those in our buttocks – are not working very well, the muscles in our back take over the task of keeping our back straight. But using the back muscles to keep the body upright proves

LIFTING A HEAVY OBJECT

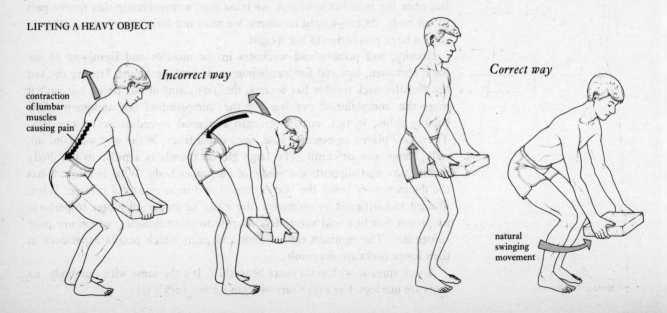

Incorrect way

contraction
of lumbar
muscles
causing pain

Correct way

natural
swinging
movement

harmful in the long run, and it is much better to keep the buttock muscles in good order so that they will work properly. We should use our leg muscles and joints to raise ourselves upright, for this is a natural body movement which causes no harm to the lumbar region.

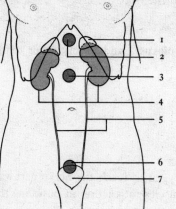

1   adrenal gland
2   solar plexus
3   upper intestinal   ⎫   serving the kidneys
     plexus   ⎭   and the adrenal glands
4   kidneys
5   ureters (between kidneys and bladder)
6   plexus of the lower abdomen:
     serving the bladder
7   bladder

/ *Exercises for relief*

As far as possible, avoid standing during attacks of pain.

1   To soothe the abdomen

Quite often the abdominal organs will be tender or sore to touch. A large part of our nerve impulses run to waste here, creating a nervous imbalance that can prevent proper co-ordination of the muscles in the lumbar region.

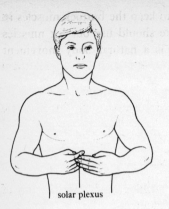

solar plexus

Place the fingers of one hand over the fingers of the other at the top of your abdomen under the point of your sternum, leaning slightly forward in a sitting or standing position.

● apply steady pressure; exhale
● maintain the pressure and breathe shallowly
● release the pressure gradually; inhale
● repeat the exercise 10 times
● give the same treatment to the other plexuses and to any other tender area in the abdomen.

2 To improve respiration

These exercises allow a better supply of oxygen to reach the nerve pathways and muscles. They bring the respiratory muscles into action in positions that are comfortable for the back, thereby relaxing the lumbar region.

Breathing exercise using the legs

Bend your knees up to your stomach and hold your legs with your hands.

● lightly squeeze your abdomen by bringing your knees up to it, thus stretching your back; exhale
● maintain the pressure and breathe shallowly

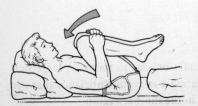

- release the pressure gently, returning your legs to their original position with your hands to prevent any jerky movement; inhale
- repeat the exercise 10 times.

Take care always to keep your legs bent over your abdomen. Stretching them makes the pain worse.

VARIATION: Bend one leg and support it with a cushion; then do the same with the other leg.

Breathing exercise using the arms

Bend your knees, supporting your legs with a cushion, and raise the top of your body if possible, with your hands on your abdomen.

- bring your arms together over your head, after describing an arc around each side of your body; inhale
- clasp your hands together above your head, stretch upwards and completely fill your lungs; inhale deeply
- bend your elbows and bring your hands back to your abdomen, passing them in front of you; exhale
- repeat the exercise 10 times.

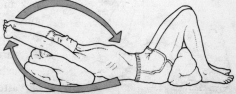

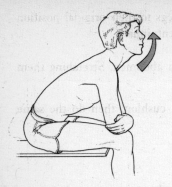

Breathing exercise using the chin

Sit down with your back rounded and your elbows folded on your knees.
- raise your chin while stretching your back; inhale
- feel the whole of your back stretching
- bring your chin back to a neutral position; exhale
- repeat the exercise 10 times.

3 To improve circulation

An improved blood supply to the lower back helps to make all the muscle and joint receptor nerves less jumpy, and relaxes tensed-up muscles. This in turn relieves the pressure exerted by the vertebrae on top of each other.

Lie flat on the floor on your back, with your legs bent and your feet supported against a wall, then slide your right hand under the base of your back and rest the other hand on the ground at an angle of 90 degrees to your body.
- gently rock your legs to the left without moving your feet; inhale
- turn over on to your right hand, compressing your back in this area; exhale
- after a series of 10 movements, reverse the procedure for the other side.

Sit on a chair and place both fists either side of your back, and against the chair.
- let yourself go backwards against your fists; inhale
- maintain the pressure; breathe shallowly
- come forward again; exhale
- repeat the movement 10 times, moving down.

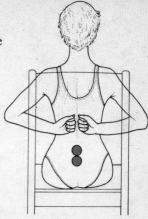

4 To relax and loosen up

Most of these exercises should be done in rotation.

Relaxing

Sit on a chair and lean well forward and to the left. Place your hands on the inside of your thighs near the knees, and open your legs wide; push your right hand against the inside of your right thigh, twisting your trunk to the left.
- slightly accentuate the twisting movement; exhale
- relax where you are; inhale
- after a series of 10 movements, reverse the procedure for the other side.

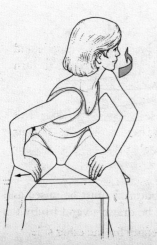

Loosening up

This is similar to the last exercise, but you breathe out while your body is being twisted, and breathe in while it is returning to its central position.

Relaxing

Kneel down, stretching out your arms in front of you, with your forehead touching the ground and your buttocks thrust to the rear.

- accentuate the movement of your buttocks by bringing them down towards your heels; exhale
- relax where you are; inhale
- repeat the procedure 10 times.

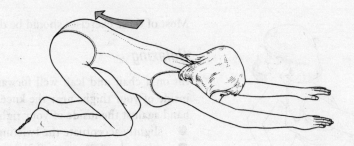

Loosening up

This exercise is similar to the last one, but your buttocks must be raised and lowered in a larger movement. Your forehead will be drawn to and fro by the movement.

Relaxing

Lie on your back and bend your left leg over your right leg, which is bent on the ground; stretch your right arm out perpendicularly to your body and look up to the ceiling.

- extend your left foot out to stretch your leg; inhale
- let your foot return to its place; exhale
- after a series of 10 movements, reverse the procedure for the other side.

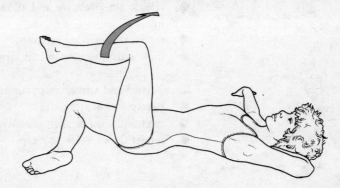

Loosening up

This exercise can strengthen the muscles and joints, and is similar to the previous one. Breathe in while extending your leg and breathe out as you bring it back to a neutral position.

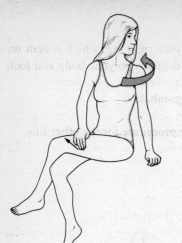

// *Stretching exercises*

1 The back muscles

Sitting on a chair, rest your left leg on your right leg; then press your right hand against your left thigh, twisting your trunk to the left.
- ● exhale as you twist your body
- ● release the pressure and allow your body to return to a neutral position; inhale
- ● repeat the exercise 10 times
- ● then make the movements larger.

Kneel down and stretch out your arms in front of you.
- ● stretch one arm; inhale
- ● stretch the other arm; exhale
- ● repeat the exercise 10 times.

Note: Do not move your buttocks or your knees (it is like walking on the spot with your hands).

2   The muscles of the abdomen

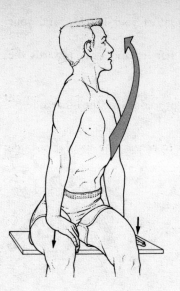

These exercises involve the often neglected transverse and oblique abdominal muscles, which are particularly important in maintaining a good posture.

Twist your trunk from a sitting position, with your right hand supported on the inner thigh and your left hand resting on the seat.
● push down and stretch up, as though trying to make yourself taller; inhale
● relax while maintaining this position; exhale
● after a series of 10 movements, reverse the procedure for the other side.

Lie down in a neutral position with your fingers interlocking above your head.
● bend your legs and rock them to the right, keeping your feet on the ground; at the same time stretch your arms upwards to the left; inhale
● return to the middle 'line of the body; exhale
● after a series of 10 movements, reverse the procedure for the other side.

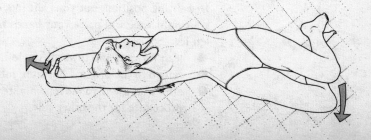

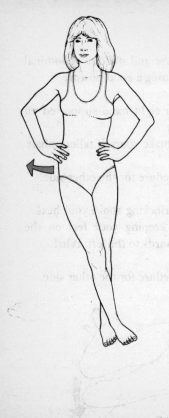

Stand against a wall with your right leg in front of your left leg, and your hands on your hips.

● take the weight of your body on to your left leg and sway towards the right; inhale
● return to the original position; exhale
● after a series of 10 movements, reverse the procedure for the other side.

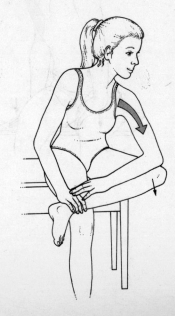

3   The leg muscles

These exercises particularly strengthen the large gluteal muscle, which can very often be stiff.

In a sitting position, put your left foot on to your right knee and place your hands on your left leg.

● lean forward and towards the left; exhale
● return to the original position; inhale
● after a series of 10 movements, reverse the procedure for the other side.

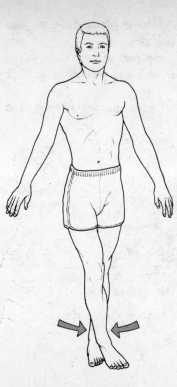

Stand up, with your legs crossed and your feet together.
- squeeze your feet and knees together; inhale
- relax; exhale
- after a series of 10 movements, reverse the
  procedure for the other side.

Lie down, cross your right leg over your left leg and put your hands on your knees.
- bend both legs and bring them up to your abdomen; exhale, and feel your right buttock stretching
- relax; inhale
- after a series of 10 movements, reverse the procedure
  for the other side.

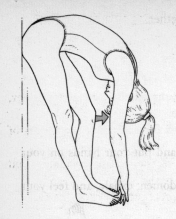

Stand up in a neutral position and gradually slide your hands down to your knees, to finish up leaning over with your arms swinging.

- slightly bend your left knee and swing the top part of your body to the left; exhale, and feel the right side of your back and your right buttock stretching
- return to the central line; inhale, and feel your muscles relaxing and loosening up
- after a series of 10 movements, reverse the procedure for the other side.

Support yourself by holding on to the uprights of a door-frame at chest height, with your feet about 3 feet away from it.

- push your buttocks backwards while holding on to the door-frame with your hands
- slightly bend your left knee, feeling the stretching along your right side; inhale
- after a series of 10 movements, reverse the procedure for the other side.

BE CAREFUL
Take care when standing upright again: at the end of the two exercises squat down. Place your hands on your knees and raise yourself by pushing down on your hands.

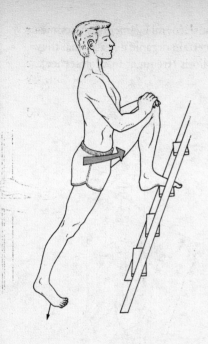

4 The very best exercise for easing and strengthening the lumbar region: one side (loin, abdomen, leg) relaxes while the other (loin, abdomen, leg) works

Stand up, with your left leg bent, and place your left foot on a stepladder, table or chair; place your hands on your left knee.

● raise yourself up on to the tip of your right foot, bringing the weight of your body forwards; exhale

● return to the starting position by pushing on your left foot; inhale – you will have a feeling of rocking from one foot to the other

● after a series of 10 movements, reverse the procedure for the other side.

Pains in the middle of the back

These are just as common and as painful as pains in the lumbar region, and are often associated with pain in the neck and shoulders. People who work in fixed positions, bent over, are well acquainted with them. The pain fluctuates between the head and the back, and may suddenly disappear in one area only to reappear in another. It sometimes reaches as far down as the lumbar region, travelling the length of the dorsal muscles. Any strong emotion or stress will make the pain worse.

These back pains are usually a result of weak muscles and ligaments, sometimes associated with arthritis in the back. Apart from certain organic diseases that they might indicate, they can be caused by kyphoscoliosis (frequent in adolescence).

/ *Exercises for relief*

1   To improve respiration

Start with your arms by your sides.
● bring your arms above your head; inhale

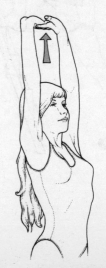

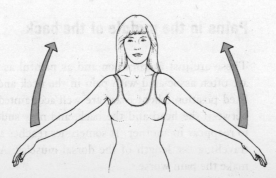

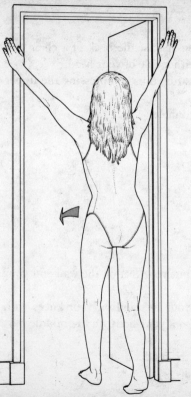

- continue to breathe in while you stretch up, with your fingers interlocked
- when you cannot breathe in any more, exhale while bringing your arms down in front of you, relaxed and half bent
- repeat the movement 10 times.

Stand up, with your arms stretched out and your hands resting on the frame of a door; then put one foot in front of the other.

- slightly bend the leg that is further back, to expand your chest and bring your back upright; inhale
- return to the starting position by stretching your front leg; exhale
- after a series of 10 movements, reverse the procedure for the other side.

VARIATION: Do the exercise in the same position, against the corner of a room.

2   To improve circulation

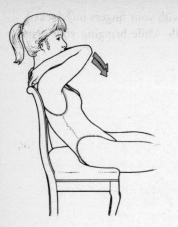

Sit down, with the back of your neck resting against the back of a chair and your hands holding the back of the chair on either side of your head.

● bring your elbows forwards and downwards, thus compressing the upper part of your back; exhale
● relax and return to the starting position; inhale
● repeat the exercise 10 times.

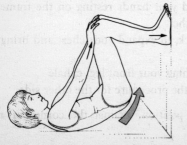

Lie down with your buttocks against a wall; put your feet on the wall and your hands on your knees.

● push simultaneously on the wall with your feet and on your knees with your hands so that you exert pressure from your body on the middle part of your back; inhale
● hold the position for a few moments on the tender areas
● lower your buttocks to the ground; exhale
● repeat the exercise 10 times.

3 Relaxing and loosening up

Put your hands on your thighs, with your fingers pointing inwards, your body half leaning forwards and your arms half bent.

To relax

Bend well forward, turning to the left.
- accentuate the twist by pushing on your right hand; exhale, and feel the stretching along your right side
- relax in this position; inhale
- after a series of 10 movements, reverse the procedure for the other side.

To loosen up

This exercise is similar to the last one, but this time lean well forward.
- push your right hand to turn your trunk to the left; exhale
- relax and return to the starting position; inhale
- after a series of 10 movements, reverse the procedure for the other side.

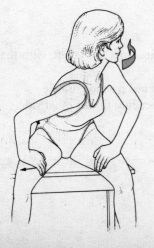

The following exercises are for the area between the shoulder-blades and their muscles; your right hand is placed over the base of your neck, while your left hand takes hold of the right elbow.

To relax

- bring your right elbow well to the left with the help of your left hand
- accentuate the movement of your right elbow towards the left; exhale
- relax in this position; inhale
- after a series of 10 movements, reverse the procedure for the other side.

To loosen up

Let your right elbow relax in front of you.

- pull your right elbow in a sweeping movement across to the left, with the help of your left hand; exhale
- relax and let your right elbow return to its original position; inhale
- after a series of 10 movements, reverse the procedure for the other side.

// *Strengthening exercises*

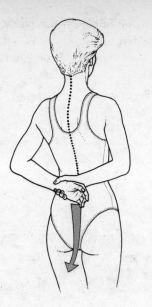

Put your hands behind your back and take hold of your left wrist with your right hand.
- stretch your arms while pulling your left wrist downwards as far as possible – this action straightens your back and expands your chest; inhale
- relax; exhale
- after a series of 10 movements, reverse the procedure for the other side.

Put your hands behind your back and let your left hand take hold of your right wrist.
- bring your right wrist to the left by pulling it with your left hand; inhale
- relax and bring your right wrist back to the starting position; exhale
- after a series of 10 movements, reverse the procedure for the other side.

Lean against a table, with your legs half bent, the palms of your hands on the edge of the table, your arms half bent and your shoulders raised.

●   push on the table with your hands to make your shoulders drop – this arches your back and expands your chest; inhale
●   relax and return to the starting position; exhale
●   repeat the exercise 10 times.

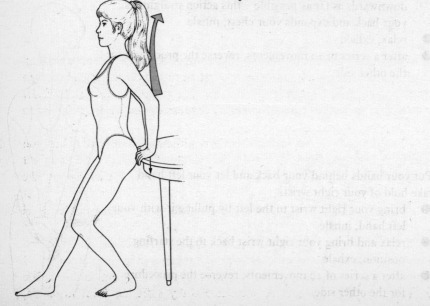

INSOMNIA AND FEELING TIRED WHEN YOU WAKE UP IN THE MORNING

You're tired and you want to go to sleep, so you close your eyes and wait. You turn on to your side, on to your stomach and on to your back. Then you turn on to your side again . . . but it's impossible: you just can't get to sleep. Now you start getting worked up and worried. Exhausted, you finally drop off to sleep, but you sleep very badly.

On the other hand, you may go to sleep without any difficulty, but you suddenly and inexplicably wake up in the middle of the night and can't get back to sleep again – or only after trying desperately for what seems like hours. Sometimes you go to sleep without any problem, but you wake up at first light and can't get any more sleep. And when you get up, you don't feel that you've had a decent rest.

If they occur only occasionally, these forms of insomnia are not too alarming, but when they become frequent and regular, they bring on a state of acute fatigue and a tendency to drowsiness and poor concentration during the day. There are also those who, without actually suffering from insomnia, complain of not having had enough sleep and find it difficult to get going in the morning, despite a ritual of coffee-drinking.

Sleep is a period of physiological rest. It is as indispensable for our body as air and water, and any shortfall in our sleep leads to troublesome irregularities in the functioning of our body.

Sometimes the cause of insomnia is clear enough. We may have an acute pain – toothache or sciatica, for example – or perhaps a heart or respiratory problem; we may abuse stimulants (tea, coffee, alcohol, tobacco); or we may complain of having 'cold feet and a hot head' (a circulatory disorder). Some minor causes of sleeplessness are preventable: for example, an evening meal that was too heavy, a bedroom which is too hot or too cold, physical or mental stress, or an ill-suited programme of nightwork. More troublesome is the short night's sleep of older people that is almost physiological. But very often insomnia is due to an imbalance in the autonomic nervous system, the result of preoccupations and worries of varying intensity, which get magnified and keep us awake in spite of ourselves – a vicious circle.

Sleeping tablets may help, but they upset the balance between the slow and rapid (dream) stages of sleep which is essential for good quality rest. To perform our waking activities to the best of our ability, we must be able to spend a third of our life at rest. It is as important to prepare ourselves for a good night's sleep as it is to plan a programme for our waking life. This extra attention to our bodies will have a positive effect upon the whole of our life.

/ *Exercises for relief*

1   To calm a state of cerebral hyperactivity

A state of cerebral hyperactivity is frequently connected with a state of tense and prolonged tightening up of the facial muscles and of the tiny scalp muscles. We are often so used to it that we don't pay it any attention.

The 'cerebral cartography' transmitted to the head and face, both from a sensory and a motor point of view, is, together with that of the hand, the most important in the body. In other words, every major activity of the face, the scalp and the hands results in corresponding activity in the brain. This treatment aims to relax the face, scalp and hands, so as to reduce cerebral excitement and induce sleep.

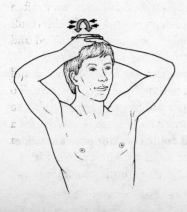

To relax the face and the scalp

Place your hands, with your fingers interlocked, on the top of your head.
- raise your scalp by bringing the palms of your hands together; inhale
- relax; exhale
- repeat the exercise 10 times
- repeat the exercise along a central line, then over the whole of your scalp.

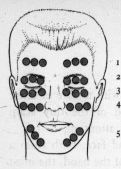

With the first three fingers of both hands, with small vertical movements to and fro, make your scalp and its muscles slide over the bone.

● repeat the exercise 10 times in each of the following areas:
1. along your forehead
2. just under your brows
3. along the lower edges of your eye-sockets
4. under your cheek-bones
5. on your chin
6. in the hollows of your temples
7. above your jaw-bone, in front of your ear
8. under the occipital bone at the back of your neck.

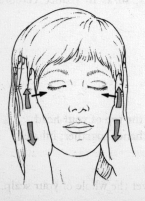

To reduce sensitivity to noise

Put the palms of your hands over your ears, and apply constant pressure while keeping your eyes closed.

● work your hands in small movements up and down until your ears grow warm.

Put your palms flat over your ears with the fingers pointing to the rear.
- apply pressure on your ears; exhale
- relax the pressure; inhale
- repeat the exercise 10 times.

In this way you induce a state of beneficial calm.

To reduce tension in the arms, and especially in the hands

Interlock the fingers of both hands in front of your chest, with your arms bent.
- stretch your arms in front of you, turning the palms outwards; exhale, and feel your fingers, hands, wrists, and arms stretching
- bring your hands back in front of your chest by bending your arms; inhale
- repeat the exercise 10 times.

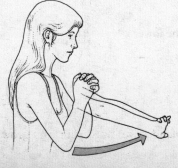

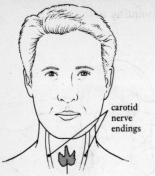

carotid nerve endings

thyroid gland

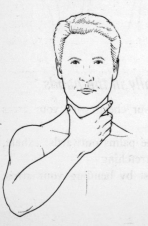

2   To calm cardiac hyperactivity

We are sometimes aware of an increase in the heart rhythm which makes it difficult to go to sleep. At the same time our blood-pressure can be slightly higher than normal.

Two avenues of treatment are possible. By applying pressure to the autonomic carotid nerve endings (receptors) and to the thyroid gland in the neck, you can induce a slowing down of the heart rhythm and a lowering of blood-pressure. The same results can be achieved by light pressure of the eyeballs.

Place one hand around the front of your neck.
- apply gentle pressure with the palm of your hand; exhale
- maintain the pressure; breathe shallowly
- gradually relax the pressure; inhale.

Lie down; using your fingers, lightly massage the lower parts of your eyeballs with your eyelids closed, breathing naturally.
- apply gentle pressure carefully
- release the pressure
- repeat the procedure 10 times
- repeat, gently massaging the upper parts of your eyeballs with your fingers.

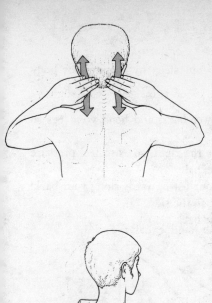

3   To relieve tension in the neck and shoulders

Place the first three fingers of both hands over the back of your neck, just at the base of the skull, on the points where your muscles are tense and tender, and apply pressure with your fingers.

● with your fingers stretch the skin and the underlying flesh downwards; inhale; feel your head being carried backwards
● with your fingers bring the muscles back to the starting position; exhale
● repeat the procedure 10 times.

Place your head in the neutral position, then bend your left arm and rest your left hand on your left side; put your right hand over your left shoulder, with your fingers curled round the bony ridge of your shoulder-blade, where the trapezius muscle is attached.

● slightly lower your right elbow – this stretches the muscle at the point where it enters the bone and makes your head turn; exhale
● bring your elbow back to the starting position; inhale
● repeat the procedure 10 times
● work in the same manner all along the ridge and the inside corner of your shoulder-blade, where the levator muscle is attached and is usually tense.
● finish with the area between your shoulder-blade and your spinal column to reach the deeper muscles
● reverse the procedure for the other side.

4 To relieve tension in the back

Tensed-up and aching muscles often disturb our sleep by keeping our body constantly on the move.

Lie down with your right fist under your lower back, and bend your legs so that your feet are flat on the floor.

- lightly rock your legs to the left, then to the right, so as to feel pressure on your lower back from your right fist; exhale
- repeat the movement, steadily moving your fist upwards along your back; inhale each time you bring your legs over to the side
- exhale each time you feel pressure in your back.

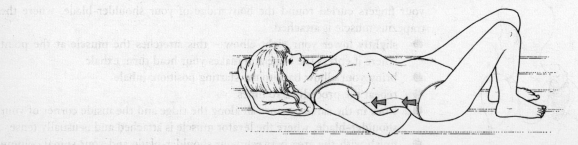

VARIATION: Do the exercise in a sitting position, with your fist between your back and the back of a chair.

5   To relieve possible digestive upsets

Heaviness in the digestive tract after too large a meal can make it difficult to sleep. First of all operate on the plexuses of your abdomen, then on the areas where you feel discomfort. (See *Digestive pains in the abdomen*, pp. 216–20.)

6   To slow down the breathing rhythm

It is difficult to go to sleep if your breathing is not calm and free from any kind of blockage or tightness.

Cross your hands over your abdomen.
- slightly inflate your abdomen; inhale as deeply as possible
- stop breathing for a few moments
- deflate your abdomen;
  exhale.

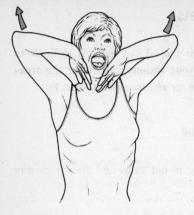

Bend and raise your elbows with the backs of your hands against your cheeks; open your mouth wide and make yourself yawn.

● accentuate the movements of your elbows upwards and to the rear; inhale
● gently relax your arms and shallowly breathe
● repeat the exercise 10 times
● bring your elbows down to a neutral position; exhale slowly.

// *Strengthening exercises*

1 **For reducing tension in the back of the neck,** see pp. 81–2.

2 **For reducing tension and pain in the back,** see pp. 89–108.

3 **For reducing anxiety,** see pp. 251–7.

RESPIRATORY PROBLEMS

Chronic bronchitis

The chief characteristic of this condition is an ordinary cough which produces bronchial secretion. It generally lasts for three months of the year. Smoking, industrial pollution or one's place of work are the main causes. It is just the opportunity that respiratory infections are looking for; eventually, permanent damage to the bronchioles makes breathing more and more difficult, and this in turn has unfortunate repercussions for the heart and lungs.

Normal exhalation is quite a passive activity, but in a case of chronic bronchitis the diameter of the bronchial tubes is reduced, and they become blocked with an abnormal amount of bronchial secretion. This means that breathing out becomes painful, eased only by coughing up phlegm. In addition, the lungs are constricted within a chest which cannot expand properly. The sufferer's back is often bent and his neck sunk into hunched shoulders.

The following are also useful for breathlessness due to a sedentary life:
- training in breathing, particularly breathing out
- exercises which expand the chest and make it work better.

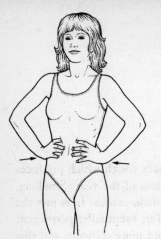

/ *Exercises for relief*

1 To improve exhalation

Work on your respiratory muscles – in particular the abdominal muscles, the diaphragm and the intercostals – by practising extended exhalation. Keep your mouth half open and breathe out through your lips, as though whistling.

Abdominal muscles

Put your hands on your hips, between your pelvis and your lowest ribs.
● press against your sides while exhaling
● maintain the pressure and breathe shallowly
● relax; inhale
● repeat the exercise 10 times.

Diaphragm muscle

Put your hands on your lowest ribs.
● apply careful pressure (so as not to damage your ribs) while exhaling
● maintain the pressure; breathe shallowly
● relax; inhale
● repeat the exercise 10 times.

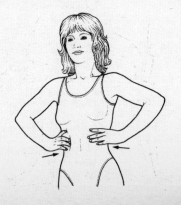

Intercostal muscles

Encircle your ribs with both hands some way down from your armpits.
- apply pressure with care while exhaling
- maintain the pressure; breathe shallowly
- relax; inhale
- repeat the exercise 10 times.

General breathing exercise

Sit down and put your hands on your knees with your legs apart.
- bend forwards so as to bring your head between your legs; exhale, emptying your lungs completely
- hold your breath for a moment
- return to a sitting position; inhale
- repeat the exercise 10 times.

2   To improve the expansion and flexibility of the chest

The aim of these exercises is to straighten your back and expand your shoulders and chest.

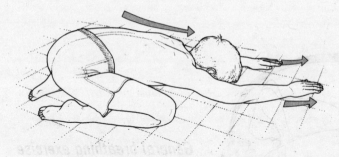

Kneel down with your buttocks on your heels; put your chin forwards on the floor with your arms stretched out in front.

● stretch one arm out in front of you, keeping your body where it is; inhale
● stretch your other arm; exhale
● repeat the exercise 10 times.

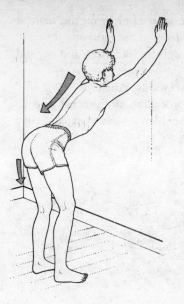

Face a wall and place the palms of your hands against it, level with your eyes; place your feet a little apart about 3 feet from the wall.

- bend your knees and feel your arms, shoulders and back stretching; inhale
- raise your chin at the same time to let more air into your lungs
- straighten your legs and your back; exhale
- repeat the exercise 10 times.

Lean back against a table, with your legs partially bent; place the palms of your hands on the edge of the table, with your arms half bent and your shoulders raised.

- push on the table with your hands to stretch your arms – this straightens your back and expands your chest; inhale
- relax and return to the starting position; exhale
- repeat the exercise 10 times.

(*Note:* you can start with your arms more bent.)

VARIATION: Use a similar stance, with your arms on a chair.

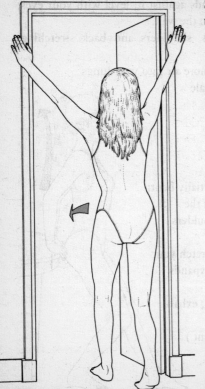

Stretch out your arms and put your hands on a door-frame or on the walls at the corner of a room; then place your left foot in front of the right one.

- slightly bend your left knee – this will straighten your back and expand your chest; inhale
- stretch your left knee to move your body backwards; exhale
- after a series of 10 movements, reverse the procedure for the other side
- repeat the exercise, placing your hands rather higher so as to expand your chest as much as possible.

// *Strengthening exercises*

See the strengthening exercises described for *Asthma*, pp. 130–32.

Asthma

This is characterized by attacks of difficult breathing (dyspoea), which mostly affect the sufferer when he is breathing out. Asthma often occurs at night. The condition is the result of a malfunction of the trachea and the bronchi due to a variety of irritants, to psychological factors, or to infections or endocrinal irregularities. The characteristic spasms of the bronchial muscles are associated with hypersecretion of the bronchi. The bronchial tubes become blocked, resulting in 'wheezing' followed by the expectoration of small drops of whitish spittle. Between attacks a normal breathing rhythm returns, but the condition can deteriorate and produce a permanent respiratory problem.

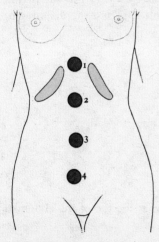

1 solar plexus
2 upper intestinal plexus
3 lower intestinal plexus
4 plexus of the lower abdomen

/ *Exercises for relief*

Even though during attacks some form of medical treatment is the first consideration, it is possible to shorten a bout of difficult breathing with exercises.

1   To relieve tension in the abdomen

Normal breathing is a passive phenomenon using the flexibility of the chest. During asthma attacks you should practise prolonged exhalation, exercising all the muscles used for breathing out in order to expel the bad air trapped in the lungs. In this way, by calming the tension which is always present in the abdomen, you make better use of the abdominal muscles and the diaphragm, which are used most in breathing out.

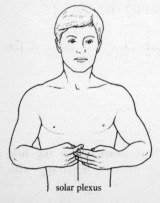

solar plexus

To treat the solar plexus

Place the fingers of one hand on those of the other at the top of the abdomen under the point of the sternum.
- increase pressure gently; exhale
- maintain the pressure and breathe shallowly
- release the pressure gradually; inhale
- repeat the exercise 10 times.

Treatment under the right ribs

Hook your fingers under your right ribs.

- increase the pressure gently; exhale
- maintain the pressure and shallow breathe
- release the pressure gradually; inhale
- repeat the exercise 10 times
- do the same under your left ribs.

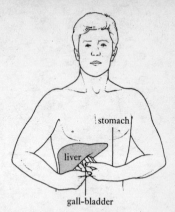

2 To improve exhalation (muscles activating the chest)

The aim here is to help the muscles used in breathing out: those of the abdomen, the diaphragm and the intercostals.

Abdominal muscles

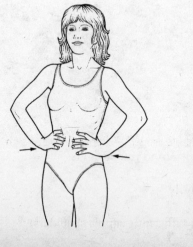

Put your hands on your hips.

- press against your sides while exhaling
- maintain the pressure and breathe shallowly
- release the pressure; inhale
- repeat the exercise 10 times.

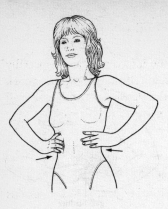

Diaphragm muscle

Put your hands on your lowest ribs.
- apply pressure carefully (without damaging your ribs) while exhaling
- maintain the pressure and breathe shallowly
- release the pressure gradually; inhale
- repeat the exercise 10 times.

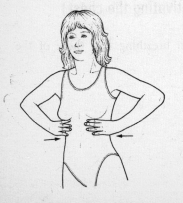

Intercostal muscles

Place your hands over your ribs some way down from your armpits.
- apply pressure carefully while exhaling
- maintain the pressure and breathe shallowly
- release the pressure gradually; inhale
- repeat the exercise 10 times (if you have sufficiently supple shoulders).

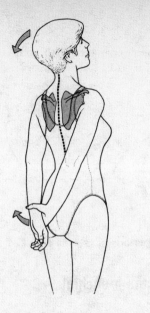

3   Improving inhalation (muscles activating the chest)

The muscles normally used in breathing in are the intercostals and especially the muscles of the diaphragm, which are contracted. During an asthma attack these are substituted by other muscles, such as the pectorals, the dorsals and the muscles of the neck. Our aim is to make these work more efficiently.

Muscles at the top of the back

With hands behind your back, grasp your left wrist with your right hand.
● stretch both arms at the same time – this will bring your shoulder-blades together; inhale
● relax; exhale
● repeat the exercise 10 times.

Muscles at the front of the neck

Place your hands, with fingers interlocked, on the crown of your head.
● at the same time, push both elbows backwards and raise the upper part of your chest with the help of the respiratory muscles in your neck; inhale
● relax; exhale
● repeat the exercise 10 times.

Pectoral muscles

Place your hands flat on a table, the width of your shoulders apart, with your buttocks well to the rear.

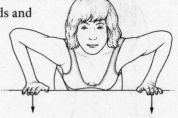

- let your chest drop on to the table; exhale
- at the same time push down on to your hands and expand the upper part of your chest with the help of your pectoral muscles; inhale
- repeat the exercise 10 times.

// *Strengthening exercises*

These are exercises to be practised exclusively *outside* periods of asthma attack.

1 To improve exhalation by making use of the bronchial muscles

[a] *Use prolonged exhalation, keeping your mouth half open and expelling the air through your lips, as in whistling.*
Place your hands flat on your knees.

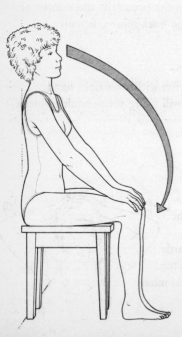

- after inhaling rather more deeply than normal, exhale slowly, leaning forwards, without inhaling again

- when you have reached the point where your head is between your legs, continue to empty your lungs completely; exhale forcibly
- sit up again; inhale
- repeat the exercise 10 times.

[b] *Use the prolonged exhalation exercise once more, but this time expel the air in short bursts. Close your mouth and nose tightly so that no air can escape in between each short exhalation.*
Use the same position as in the previous exercise.

- after inhaling rather more deeply than normal, exhale in little bursts lasting a second and close your mouth and nose tightly for a second after each burst
- when your head comes between your knees, empty your lungs completely; exhale forcibly
- sit up again while breathing in
- repeat the exercise 10 times.

[c] *Rapid exhalation exercise [to be practised after the previous two]. This exercise increases the power of the bronchial muscles to expel air.*
Get into the same position as before.

- after inhaling rather more deeply than normal, close your mouth and throat (with the glottis closed), keeping the air in your lungs, then, without releasing the air, contract your abdominal muscles and the other respiratory muscles so as to increase the pressure in your abdomen and lungs (as in straining on the toilet)

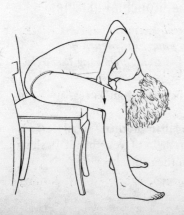

- when the pressure has been built up sufficiently, suddenly open your mouth and throat to let the air come out with an explosion; bend forward, bringing your head between your knees so that you can empty your lungs completely; exhale forcibly
- sit up again, breathe in
- repeat the exercise several times.

(*Note*: this exercise may start you coughing and upset you slightly for a while: if so, repeat the previous exercises.)

2 To improve inhalation by working the bronchial muscles

[a] *Use the prolonged inhalation exercise, keeping your mouth half open and drawing the air in through your lips* [*as though sucking through a straw*].

Bend your body well forward, with your head between your knees, and your hands on your knees.

- after breathing out rather more forcibly than normal, inhale slowly through your lips, while sitting up with the help of your hands pushing on your knees; do not exhale until you reach the neutral position
- then exhale
- repeat the exercise several times.

[*b*]   *Using the prolonged inhalation exercise, but this time breathing in the air in short gulps, keep your mouth and nose tightly closed between each mouthful of air inhaled.*

Use the same position as in the previous exercise.

● after breathing out rather more forcibly than normal, inhale in short gulps of a second's duration; and close your mouth and nose tightly for a second between each short inhalation

● after returning to the neutral position, fill your lungs with air completely

● then exhale

● repeat the exercise several times.

[*c*]   *Rapid inhalation exercise [to be practised after the previous two]. This exercise increases the ability of the bronchi to open as the air is drawn in.*

Get into the same position as in the previous exercise.

● after breathing out rather more deeply than usual, close your mouth and throat slightly (with the glottis closed); without inhaling, sit upright and remain without breathing

● raise the top part of your chest with the help of your neck muscles, so as to increase the feeling of emptiness in your lungs; push down with your hands on your thighs, with your arms stretched, to help you

● as soon as you feel that you need air, suddenly open your mouth and throat to breathe in air with a kind of explosion; throw your head and

trunk lightly backwards as you push down with your hands to help you fill your lungs completely; inhale forcibly
● then exhale
● repeat the exercise several times.

(*Note*: this exercise may start you coughing and upset you slightly for a while: if so, repeat the previous exercises.)

3   To improve muscular synchronization

The muscles which allow the expansion and contraction of the rib cage during inhalation and exhalation are all too often stiff, and this leads to a lack of synchronization with the bronchial muscles which are engaged in increasing and decreasing the diameter of the bronchi. The result is a more permanent respiratory problem.

For this situation we use, in conjunction with the techniques described earlier:
● exercises for the muscles of the rib cage, performed with
● exercises for the bronchial muscle.

[a]   *Example of a compound exercise for exhalation.*
Sit down and put your hands on your thighs.
● after breathing in rather more deeply than normal, exhale slowly, leaning forwards and squeezing your sides, without breathing in again

- when your head is between your legs, continue to empty your lungs completely, helped by pressure from your hands on your hips; exhale forcibly
- sit up again, inhaling
- repeat the exercise several times.

Put your hands on your lowest ribs and perform the same exercise. Clasp your sides under your armpits with your hands and perform the same exercise.

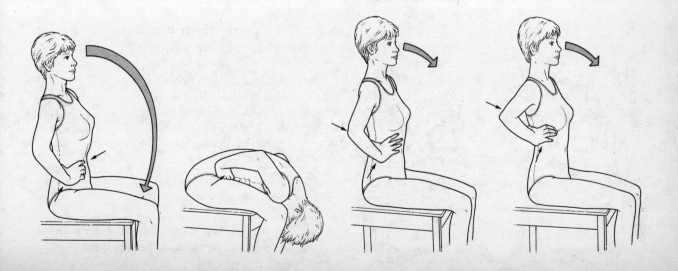

[b]   *Example of a composite exercise for inhalation.*

Sit down and put your hands behind your back, with your right hand clasping your left wrist and your body bent forwards with your head between your legs.

● after exhaling rather more completely than normal, inhale slowly as you come up and stretch both arms at the same time

● sitting in a neutral position, continue filling your lungs to their full capacity with the help of your arms stretching down behind and your shoulder-blades coming together; inhale forcibly

● then exhale

● repeat the exercise several times.

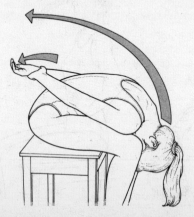

It is possible to invent other exercises along the same lines as these.

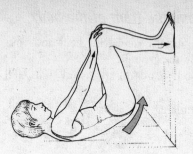

4 Improving the blood supply to the nervous pathways controlling respiration

1 *The autonomic nervous pathways in the back*

Lie with your buttocks against a wall, your feet on the wall, and your hands on your knees.

● push simultaneously on the wall with your feet and on your knees with your hands, so as to apply pressure with your body weight on the upper part of your back; inhale

● remain for a few moments with the weight on this area; breathe normally

● bring your buttocks down to the ground; exhale

● repeat the exercise several times.

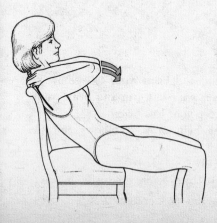

Rest the back of your neck on the top of a chair-back and grip the chair-back on either side of your head with your hands.

● bring your elbows forwards and downwards without letting go of the chair-back; this will exert pressure on the very top of your back; exhale

● maintain the pressure; breathe shallowly

● relax the pressure and let your elbows return to the starting position; inhale

● repeat the exercise 10 times.

2   *Autonomic nervous pathways along the front of the body*

Lie down on your front in a neutral position, with your arms bent and your hands level with your head; keep your chin on the ground.

- lift up your chin and push down on your hands to arch your body and expand your chest; inhale
- drop back on to the ground so as to stimulate the front part of your chest; exhale
- remain lying on the ground a few moments; breathe naturally
- repeat the exercise several times.

Grip your right shoulder with your left hand and bring your left elbow in close to your chest; place your right arm over your left arm and bring your right hand across to grip your left shoulder; keep your legs together.

- gradually squeeze your chest with the help of your elbows and by bending slightly forwards; exhale
- maintain the pressure and breathe shallowly
- as soon as you feel the need for air, release the pressure gradually; inhale
- repeat the exercise 10 times.

3   Nerves in the neck controlling the diaphragm

The nerves serving the diaphragm lie in the neck and emerge from the spinal cord at the level of the middle cervical vertebrae (third and fourth). In other words, we breathe by virtue of our neck. When the neck is contracted, these nerves are irritated and are deprived of a good circulation.

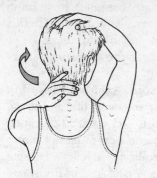

Put your right hand on your head, and curl your left hand round the projections of your middle cervical vertebrae.
● lower your left elbow, thereby stretching the back of your neck and making your head turn to the right; exhale
● raise your left elbow to make your head return; inhale
● after a series of 10 movements, reverse the procedure for the other side.

Problems caused by smoking

It all starts with those first puffs at school, which make most of us cough (a respiratory reflex). Trying to be grown-up, we feel that a 'fag' helps us become one of the group. Gradually we reach the stage where we are never without a packet of cigarettes; we would feel something was missing without them. Always at hand, in our pocket or our bag, the packet of cigarettes

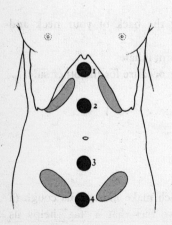

1 solar plexus
2 upper intestinal plexus
3 lower intestinal plexus
4 plexus of the lower abdomen

becomes our inseparable friend, helping us relax and soothing our nerves when we feel anxious or fed up.

If you are a reasonably healthy smoker you don't pay too much attention to anti-smoking campaigns. Chronic bronchitis, cardiovascular problems, arteritis (inflammation of the arteries) in the legs, cancer of the bronchi, the lungs or the digestive system – all these are other people's problems. Smoking relaxes you, makes you feel good . . . like coffee does.

Life's often tough: housing problems, commuting, confrontations with people, competition, unemployment, setbacks in our emotional life, and so on. These things can easily get on top of us; we begin to feel we are suffocating physically and mentally. We just can't wait to jump into a car or on to a motor bike, or . . . to have a cigarette. Without our realizing it, our exhausted nervous system calls out for a larger intake of oxygen. And, paradoxically, we smoke! In order to stimulate our respiratory system, we resort to nicotine.

Here lies the reason for the relative failure of anti-smoking campaigns in some countries. And when smoking as a means to help us unwind proves ineffective, some of us may turn to more drastic social props: one addiction can lead to another.

But what about training our lungs to function better, to achieve a better consumption of oxygen – without smoking? This vital oxygen will help us to tackle all our daily problems. We need breathing exercises and exercises which strengthen our nervous system, coupled with other methods of ridding the system of toxins. That way we will be able to give up smoking without too much difficulty – we won't have the feeling that 'something is missing'.

1 To reduce the feeling of stress in the abdomen

A feeling of stress is almost always present in our abdomen, so we must try to relax the nervous plexuses, and in particular the solar plexus and the regions beneath our lower ribs (see illustration on p. 140).

To apply pressure to the solar plexus

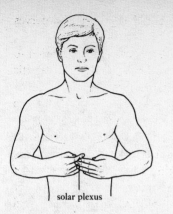

solar plexus

Put your fingers together and place them at the top of your abdomen under the point of your sternum.
- apply pressure gradually; exhale
- maintain the pressure and breathe shallowly
- gradually release the pressure; inhale deeply
- repeat the exercise 10 times
- apply the same treatment to your other plexuses and tender areas
- for the areas beneath your left and right ribs, gently penetrate beneath the ribs with your fingers.

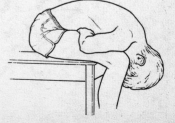

You can also lean forward with your head between your legs, bend your arms on your thighs, and put your fingers on the tender areas of your plexus.

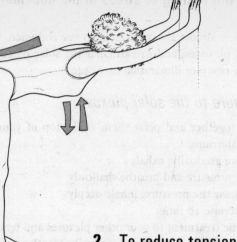

2 To reduce tension in the back and shoulders

Stand with your hands against a wall, level with your chest, and stretch out your arms; your legs should be slightly apart and stretched, and your feet placed so that your back is flat.

- let your chest fall but keep your hands in the same position; inhale, and feel your arms, shoulders and back stretching
- let your back spring back lightly; exhale
- repeat the exercise 10 times.

Sit on a chair and lean on the edge of a desk with your elbows bent and your hands on top of one another. Put your forehead on your hands; and sit well enough back on the chair to ensure that your back is stretched.

- push downwards and backwards on your elbows; exhale
- relax the pressure; inhale
- repeat the exercise 10 times.

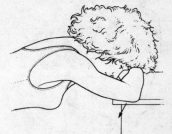

Stand with your buttocks against a wall, your legs slightly apart and stretched, and your feet about 20 inches from the wall; then lean forward, keeping your buttocks against the wall, with your arms hanging down.

- simultaneously (a) throw your right arm to the left and your right hand as close as possible to the ground, and (b) bring your bent left elbow towards your back; exhale
- bring both your arms back to the starting position; inhale
- after a series of 10 movements, reverse the procedure for the other side.

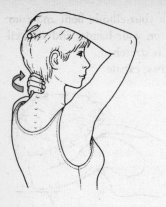

3 To stretch the back of the neck at the point through which the nerves to the diaphragm pass

Put your right hand flat on the crown of your head, with the fingers of your left hand curling round the projections of your middle neck vertebrae.

- lower your left elbow so as to stretch the back of your neck and make your head turn to the right; exhale
- lift your elbow and allow your head to return to the starting position; inhale
- after a series of 10 movements, reverse the procedure for the other side.

4 To improve chest expansion

Place the palms of your hands on a wall level with your eyes, and move backwards so that your feet are apart, about 3 feet from the wall, and your back is flat.

- slightly bend your knees while keeping your hands and feet in the same position;

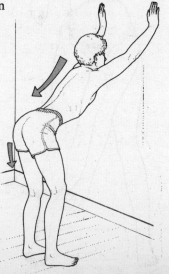

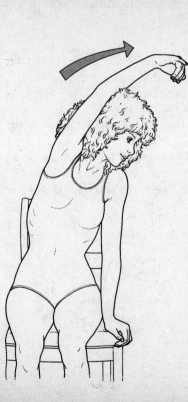

inhale deeply, and feel your arms, shoulders and back stretching; lift your chin to deepen your breathing
- stretch your legs and arch your back; exhale
- repeat the exercise 10 times.

Sit down with your left hand on the seat of your chair and your right arm above your head.
- stretch your right side by taking your right hand further to the left; inhale
- relax; exhale
- gradually increase the stretching
- when you reach the limit to which you can stretch, inhale slowly and deeply and hold your breath in for a few seconds
- after a series of 10 movements, reverse the procedure for the other side.

5   Breathing exercises

Get used to holding your breath.
● after a deep breath in
● after a deep breath out.

Sit down, with your hands on your sides under your lower ribs.
● exhale slowly while bending forwards and squeezing your sides with your hands; exhale deeply, and do not breathe in immediately
● come up again, inhaling slowly; then hold your breath for a moment
● repeat the exercise 10 times
● repeat the procedure with your hands on your lower ribs, and then with your hands under your armpits.

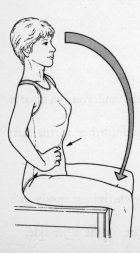

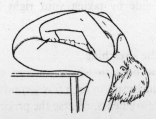

Sit down with your hands behind your back and your right hand clasping your left wrist; put your feet apart and bend your body forward with your head between your legs.

- inhale slowly and deeply while coming up and stretching your arms behind your back; completely fill your lungs with air while sitting up, and hold your breath in
- exhale slowly while bending forward to return to the starting position; then, with your head between your legs, refrain from breathing for a few seconds
- repeat the exercise 10 times.

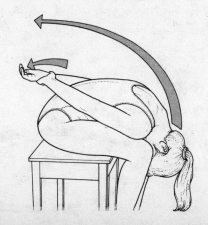

Lie down and raise your pelvis with the help of your elbows against the floor and your hands against your lower back; stretch your legs without putting excessive pressure on your neck.

- exhale slowly and fully while lowering your legs a little more; refrain from breathing in for a few moments
- as soon as you feel you need air, bring your pelvis down to the ground while inhaling deeply
- continue to inhale while completely stretching your body on the ground; hold your breath for a few moments
- repeat the exercise 10 times.

Lie on a bed, a bench or two chairs side by side, either with your legs bent on the bed or with your feet placed comfortably on the floor, or if necessary on some books. Put your arms above your head and hold a 5–6 lb weight in your hands. Rest the back of your neck on the edge (use another chair if necessary) so that your head hangs back.

- take your hands nearer to the ground, with your arms relaxed; inhale deeply and hold your breath for a moment
- bring the weight back up and over your head to place it on your abdomen, while exhaling slowly; refrain from breathing in for a moment
- repeat the exercise 10 times.

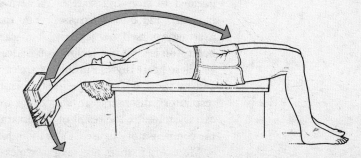

For relieving stress, see *Stress*, pp. 258–64.

PROBLEMS WITH HEART RHYTHM

Extrasystoles

You have a feeling that your heart has missed a beat; that it has suddenly decided to stop and start of its own accord. You feel dazed or dizzy for a moment, and quite distressed. You can't understand why: you haven't been exerting yourself particularly. You can't help getting worried. To feel your heart stop is a bit like feeling you're dead!

These heart rhythm problems are experienced by anxious or nervous people, and by those who indulge in stimulants of one kind or another. Digestive or respiratory disorders can also bring them on. What happens exactly? These extrasystoles are the result of a premature contraction of the heart, followed by the compensatory pause. It's as though the heart has made a little mistake.

More often than not, extrasystoles are not of a pathological nature. It's reassuring to note that they disappear with physical effort – if they *occurred* with physical effort one might suspect a cardiac problem. They are caused by an imbalance in the autonomic nervous system, and if they occur frequently they can give rise to a feeling of permanent anxiety. It's a good idea to have a medical examination in any case.

I *Exercises for relief*

1 To improve the digestion

Flatulence or difficult digestion after a meal can often produce extrasystoles.

If you have spasms and flatulence in your digestive tract, use slowly applied pressure. Apply pressure with a rapid rhythm in the case of sluggish digestion. Always start with slowly applied pressure.

To exert pressure on the solar plexus

Put your fingers together, so that those of one hand are on top of those of the other, then place them at the top of your abdomen under the point of your sternum.

- apply pressure, increasing it steadily; exhale
- maintain a constant pressure and breathe shallowly
- gradually release the pressure; inhale
- repeat the exercise 10 times.

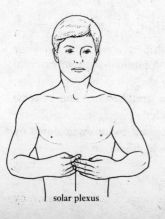

solar plexus

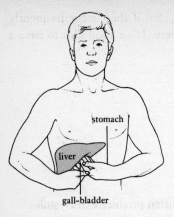

To exert pressure beneath the ribs

Hook your fingers under your right ribs.
- apply pressure gently, penetrating beneath the ribs with your fingers; exhale
- maintain the pressure, breathing shallowly
- release the pressure gradually; inhale – this treats the liver and the gall-bladder
- after a series of 10 applications, reverse the procedure for the other side – this treats the stomach.

Apply the same treatment to any other tender area of your abdomen.

2   To improve respiration and heart function

This exercise allows us to apply a 'chest massage' combined with an external heart massage, resulting in improved respiration.

Lie face downwards on the floor with your arms stretched out and bent on either side of your head and your chin on the ground.
- slowly raise your chin upwards towards the ceiling by pushing down on your hands, without arching your back too much; inhale slowly
- pause while continuing to inhale deeply
- lower your body to the ground; exhale
- repeat the exercise 10 times.

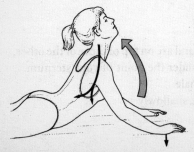

Sit down with your hands behind your back and your right hand clasping your left wrist; then bend forwards and rest your chest on your thighs, keeping your legs together.

- inhale slowly and deeply as you straighten up and stretch your arms behind your back; fill your lungs completely as you sit up and hold your breath in
- let your chest drop down to your thighs again and feel some pressure; exhale
- repeat the exercise 10 times.

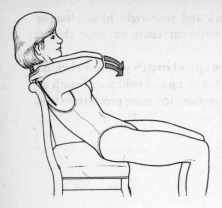

3 To improve the blood supply to the autonomic nervous pathways of the back

Sit on a chair and rest the back of your neck on the chair-back, with your hands gripping the chair-back on each side of your head.

● bring your elbows forwards and downwards, without letting go of the chair – this will produce pressure on the very top of your back; exhale
● maintain the pressure and breathe shallowly
● release the pressure and let your elbows come back upwards again; inhale
● repeat the exercise 10 times.

// ***Strengthening exercises,*** see *Anxiety*, pp. 256–7, and *Stress*, pp. 265–7.

Palpitations

All of a sudden, when you are not doing anything in particular, your heart seems to bolt like a wild horse, beating more than a hundred times a minute. You feel weak and unwell. It's difficult to breathe and you feel very distressed. Even though you don't lose consciousness, it's a very disturbing experience.

This condition can suddenly come about quite naturally while you are engaged in unaccustomed or intense physical activity. The heart is responding to a greater demand for energy by quickening its rhythm. Alternatively, people whose hearts are quite healthy but who are of an emotional or impressionable disposition may be affected: particularly stressful situations (a period of examinations or competition of some kind, for example), the abuse of stimulants (tobacco, coffee, etc.) or flatulence can bring on palpitations. Physical or nervous over-exertion is very often responsible, as the result of some disturbance of the autonomic nervous balance, but sufferers should have a medical examination.

/ *Exercises for relief*

1 To calm the digestive tract

To apply pressure to the solar plexus

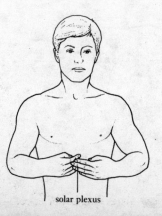

solar plexus

Place the fingers of one hand over those of the other at the top of your abdomen under the point of the sternum.
- apply pressure, increasing it steadily; exhale
- maintain a constant pressure for a few moments, breathing shallowly
- release the pressure gradually; inhale slowly
- repeat the exercise 10 times.

Treatment under the lower ribs

Hook your fingers under your right ribs.

- apply gentle pressure, penetrating with your fingers under your ribs; exhale – (this treats the liver, the gall-bladder and the large intestine)
- maintain a constant pressure for a few moments, breathing shallowly
- gradually release the pressure; inhale slowly
- after a series of 10 applications, reverse the procedure for the other side.

Apply the same treatment to every tender area of your abdomen.

2   To improve the respiration

An insufficient supply of oxygen always makes the autonomic nervous system sensitive and tends to quicken the heart rhythm. You must practise large, slow, breathing exercises to remedy the problem.

Lean forward with your hands placed at chest height for support, on a wall,

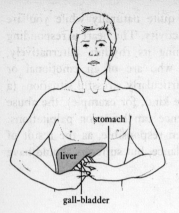

stomach

liver

gall-bladder

a piece of furniture or a door frame. Stand with your legs straight and apart so that your back is flat.

- lift your chin and head back; inhale and hold your breath for a few moments
- let your head and chin return to your chest; exhale briefly
- repeat the exercise 10 times.

This exercise helps the shoulders and hands to loosen at the same time. Place your hands, with fingers entwined, on top of your head and keep your legs together.

- stretch your arms above your head and inhale deeply
- with the palms of your hands turned upwards to the ceiling, stretch right up to your fingertips; hold your breath
- bring your hands, with your fingers still entwined, back to the top of your head; exhale
- repeat the exercise 10 times.

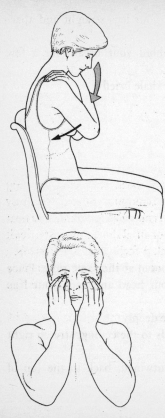

3   To calm the cardiac rhythm

Grip your right shoulder with your left hand and bring your left elbow close against your chest; bend your right arm and place it on top of your left arm. Grip your left shoulder with your right hand and keep your legs together.

- apply increasing pressure to your chest with the help of your elbows, while leaning slightly forwards; exhale
- maintain the pressure and breathe shallowly
- as soon as you feel you need air, release the pressure gradually; inhale
- repeat the exercise 10 times.

This exercise, which should be practised only in a lying position, slows down the cardiac rhythm, which might be quite fast. Place your fingers lightly on the lower part of your eye-sockets with your eyelids closed.

- breathe naturally
- apply pressure gently and carefully
- maintain the pressure for a few moments
- release the pressure
- repeat the procedure 10 times.

VARIATION: Use the palms of your hands to apply gentle pressure.

// *Strengthening exercises,* see *Anxiety*, pp. 256–7, and *Stress*, pp. 265–7.

VASOMOTOR PROBLEMS IN THE CIRCULATORY SYSTEM

Dizziness and ringing in the ears

Sometimes when you are very tired, after a heavy meal, after concentrating very hard for some time, or as a result of some intense emotion, you may feel dizzy and/or experience intermittent ringing in your ears. It may also occur during a boat or car journey, or as the result of some kind of visual or aural shock. In most cases it does not last long, and you quickly return to normal. A feeling of anxiety is often associated with these disorders and can be a further contributory factor. You may also experience dizziness when you are very hungry, or when you are suffering from insomnia or low blood-pressure.

It is advisable to have a medical check-up, in case the problem is caused by high blood-pressure.

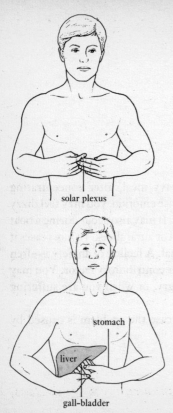

solar plexus

stomach

liver

gall-bladder

/ *Exercises for relief*

1 To calm the digestive tract

To apply pressure to the solar plexus

Place the fingers of one hand over the fingers of the other at the top of your abdomen under the point of your sternum.
- apply gentle pressure and increase it gradually; exhale
- maintain a constant pressure for a few moments; breathe shallowly
- gradually release the pressure; inhale
- repeat the exercise 10 times.
- apply the same treatment to the other plexuses of your abdomen.

To apply pressure to the area beneath the ribs

Hook your fingers under your right ribs.
- apply gentle pressure, then increase it steadily and penetrate under your ribs with your fingers; exhale
- maintain a constant pressure for a few moments; breathe shallowly
- gradually release the pressure; inhale
- after a series of 10 applications, reverse the procedure for the other side.

2 To reduce contractions and tension in the back of the neck and in the shoulders

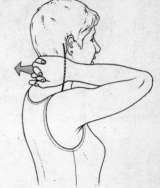

Place your hands one over the other on the back of your neck, and relax your arms.
- squeeze the muscles running up the back of your neck by bringing your palms together; exhale
- maintain the pressure; breathe shallowly
- release the pressure; inhale
- repeat the exercise 10 times
- do the same thing all along your neck.

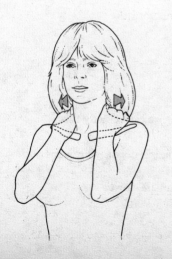

Place your hands, one on either side of your neck, at the top of your shoulders and on the trapezius muscles.
- apply pressure in the hollows above your shoulder-blades, downwards towards the trapezius muscles; exhale
- maintain the pressure; breathe shallowly
- relax; inhale
- repeat the exercise 10 times.

For other exercises, see *Tension in the back of the neck and in the shoulders*, pp. 79–85.

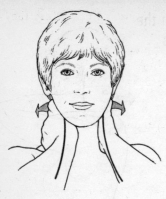

3   To improve the blood supply to the brain

This exercise operates on the autonomic nervous pathways of the neck; stimulating them causes an immediate rush of blood to the face and head through the dilated arteries.

Place the palms of both hands over the sides of your neck.
● apply gentle pressure towards the back of both sides of your neck; exhale
● maintain the pressure and breathe shallowly
● relax; inhale
● repeat the procedure 10 times.

4   To improve respiration

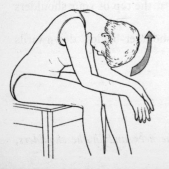

Nerve cells are sensitive to a decrease of oxygen, but we can remedy this.

Put your elbows on your knees, with your head hanging down, your arms and hands quite relaxed, and your legs apart.
● raise your chin and head up towards the rear; inhale slowly
● hold your breath for a few minutes
● return to your original position; exhale
● repeat the exercise 10 times.

Kneel down with your buttocks resting on your heels, your forehead on the ground and your arms extended forwards along the ground.

- stretch one arm, without moving your buttocks; inhale slowly
- keep your other arm quite relaxed and draw it back; exhale
- after a series of 10 movements, reverse the procedure for the other side.

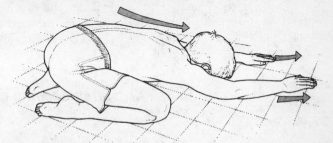

5 To reduce sensitivity to noise

Sometimes one has a feeling of exaggerated sensitivity in the ears. The following exercises will help to reduce this.

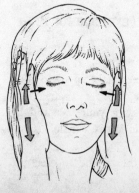

Place the palms of your hands over your ears and close your eyes.

- breathe naturally
- slide your hands gently up and down over your ears
- repeat the procedure 10 times.

Place the palms of your hands flat against your ears, with your fingers pointing backwards, and close your eyes.

● gradually increase pressure on your ears; exhale
● maintain the pressure and breathe shallowly
● release the pressure; inhale
● repeat the procedure 10 times.

// *Strengthening exercises*

1 To improve the blood supply to the brain (exercise for the abdominal muscles)

Lie down with your feet against a wall so that your knees make an angle of 90 degrees, and put your hands on your knees.

● at the same time, push lightly against the wall with your feet and by pulling on your hands bring your head towards your knees; exhale
● let your body relax on to the ground; inhale
● after repeating the exercise several times, rest on the ground and feel the blood flowing vigorously towards your head.

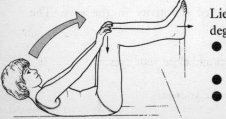

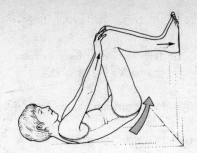

2   To improve the circulation to the whole of your autonomic nervous system

To function effectively, the nervous system must receive a good blood supply.

To improve circulation to the spinal cord

Lie down with your buttocks and feet against a wall and your hands on your knees or thighs.

- simultaneously push (a) against the wall with your feet and (b) on your knees with your hands, to raise your body gradually off the ground, starting with your lower back; inhale
- each time your body is raised inhale; each time it is lowered, exhale
- work on the whole of your back, then bring your thighs down to the floor; exhale
- repeat several times.

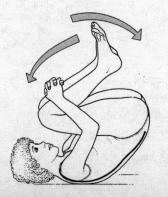

Lie on your back and grasp your knees with your hands or wrap your arms round them.

- roll backwards; exhale
- roll forwards; inhale
- work on the whole of your upper back
- repeat the exercise 10 times.

3 Respiration

Put your elbows on the ground and your hands under your lower back to raise your pelvis. Keep your legs relaxed and make sure the back of your neck is not under excessive pressure.

- breathe naturally for a few moments in this position, then exhale but do not breathe in yet
- as soon as you feel you need air, lower your pelvis to the ground as you inhale
- continue to inhale as you stretch out your body on the ground
- repeat the exercise several times.

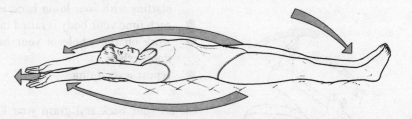

4 To reduce tension in the back of the neck and in the shoulders, see *Tension in the back of the neck and in the shoulders*, pp. 79–85.

Heaviness in the legs, varicose veins

Most of us have suffered from a heavy feeling in our legs at some time or other. If we habitually sit for long hours at a desk, in a car, on a train, or at home in front of the television screen or a computer, our legs cannot cope easily with more prolonged effort. When we settle down in a comfortable armchair to watch a film or listen to a few records or cassettes, or sit down to a well-earned meal, our mind keeps on working – it mulls over professional matters or family problems, and is stimulated by sport on the television, or adventure films – but our bodies, especially our legs, are tired.

From an initial sensation of heaviness, followed by cramps, we eventually reach a stage when we may start having trouble with varicose veins. A narrowing of the superficial veins in our legs means we easily tire when we stand up. And there may be further complications: for example, brown patches on the skin, varicose ulcers on the legs, painful attacks of phlebitis associated with the coagulation of blood in the veins. Though these conditions are fairly harmless in themselves, there is always a risk that phlebitis may turn into a more deep-seated problem, accompanied by a risk of thrombosis and pulmonary embolism.

The cause of the trouble lies in the slowing down of the return of venous blood from the legs to the heart. The blood in the deep venous system flows back to the network of veins near the surface of the leg and makes it swell up: hence the appearance of varicose veins.

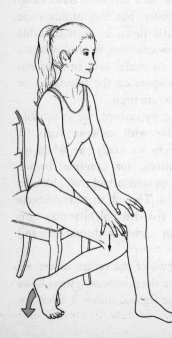

No matter how hard it tries, the heart can only pump into the arteries the amount of blood it receives. The rhythmic contraction and relaxation of our muscles, particularly those in our legs when we walk or run, cause a corresponding compression and decompression of the veins; and thanks to small valves in these veins, blood is returned to the heart along a one-way system. When we breathe in, pressure in the thorax decreases while pressure in the abdomen increases: in this way blood is drawn towards the heart. When we breathe out, the pressure in the abdomen tends to decrease and blood is drawn towards the lower limbs.

Although they do not have as many muscular fibres as the arteries, the veins can also contract under the influence of the autonomic nervous system. The impact on the veins in the soles of our feet when we walk or run at a sustained fast pace also helps to drive blood along the veins. Giving the legs and breathing mechanism plenty of work to do is essential to recuperation after illness.

/ *Exercises for relief*

1   To improve the function of the leg muscles

Sit on the edge of a chair with your hands on your knees, your left foot flat on the ground and your right foot bent and resting on the toes.

- push your right knee with your right hand, bending your right ankle more so that you can lower your right heel to the ground; inhale; feel the stretching in your right calf and the contraction along the front of your right leg
- let your knee spring back and push on your toes to raise your heel from the ground: exhale; feel the contraction in your right calf and the tension in the front of your leg
- after a series of 10 movements, reverse the procedure for the other side.

Sit down with your left foot on your right knee and your hands placed on your left leg.

- bend forwards over your left knee and push it down with your left elbow; exhale; feel the tension at the back of your left thigh (the muscles of the buttocks)
- relax; inhale
- after a series of 10 movements, reverse the procedure for the other side.

Sit down with your buttocks on the edge of a chair. Stretch your arms, holding on to the seat of the chair to the rear, and stretch your legs out in front, one on top of the other.

● stretch your legs hard and squeeze together your feet, knees, thighs and buttocks; inhale
● stretch your body slightly backwards to help you breathe in more deeply
● relax; exhale
● reverse the position of your legs and repeat the exercise.

Lie down some distance from a wall so that your legs are slightly bent and your feet are against the wall; relax your arms on the floor with your hands on your abdomen.

● push on the wall first with one foot and then with the other
● inhale on the 2nd and 3rd 'step' and exhale on the 1st
● repeat the exercise *ad lib*.

2   To improve the respiration

Lie with your buttocks against a wall or at a distance of 12–15 inches away from it, and put your hands on your knees.
- bring your knees up to your chest; exhale, expelling all the air from your lungs
- slide your feet up the wall and stretch your legs with the help of both hands pushing down on them: inhale, completely filling your lungs while pushing as hard as possible on your arms and bringing your chin in towards your chest
- repeat the exercise 10 times.

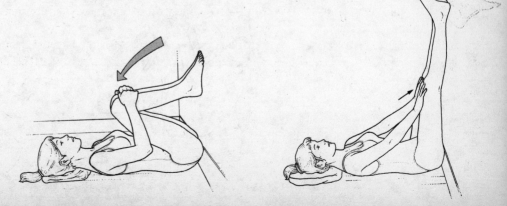

Sit on the front of a chair with your legs together and your hands on your knees.

● bring your knees up to your chest and rock back against the back of the chair; exhale
● bring your legs down to the ground with your feet flat on the floor, and sit up straight by pushing down on your stretched arms and stretching the back of your neck; inhale deeply
● repeat the exercise 10 times.

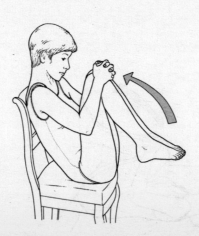

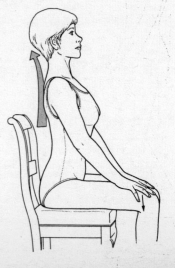

// *Strengthening exercises*

1   To improve the functioning of the arm muscles

Stand with your back against a wall (for greater stability), and place your feet slightly apart about 8 inches from the wall.
- rise up on tip-toe; inhale
- drop back to the ground without letting your back leave the wall; exhale
- repeat the exercise 10 times.

VARIATION 1: Jump on the spot.
- on every 2nd and 3rd jump inhale
- on every 1st jump exhale.

VARIATION 2: Run on the spot.
- on every 2nd and 3rd step inhale
- on every 1st step exhale.

Squat down with your hands on the ground.

● push down on your feet and stretch your legs while keeping your hands on the ground; inhale deeply
● bring your buttocks down to your heels; exhale
● repeat the exercise 10 times.

VARIATION: Use the same movements, but with your hands on a chair.

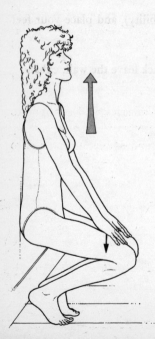

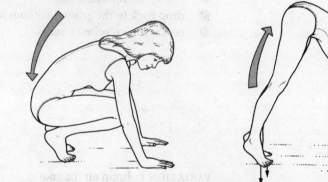

Squat down with your back against a wall and your hands on your knees.
● pushing on your knees, stand up and slide your back up the wall; inhale deeply
● return to the starting position by sliding your back down the wall; exhale
● repeat the exercise 10 times.

2   Respiration and circulation

Lie down on the ground with your feet against a wall and your arms lying along your body.

- stretch out your arms and slide them along the floor until they are behind your head; inhale slowly
- with your arms above your head, entwine the fingers of both hands and continue to inhale while stretching the top half of your body
- bring your bent arms, with the fingers still entwined, down in front of your chest and exhale slowly
- use the movement to contract your abdominal muscles, and continue to exhale as much as possible as you bring your head towards your knees
- return to the ground, separating your fingers and sliding your arms to your sides to repeat the exercise
- repeat the exercise 10 times

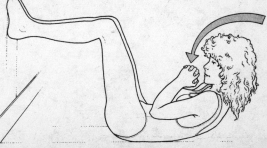

Sit down with your legs together and put your hands round the back of your neck with your fingers entwined.

- push your elbows a little further back; inhale
- stretch your arms up, turning the palms upwards; continue to inhale
- hold your breath for a few moments
- bend your elbows and squeeze your arms against your chest; exhale
- repeat the exercise 10 times.

'Pins and needles' and numbness in the fingers

Cold weather, strong emotion or menstrual periods can produce these symptoms in the fingers (sometimes in the feet and more rarely in the nose and ears). The extremities become white, starved of blood and painful, then after a few minutes everything returns to normal. If the attack lasts longer, a local deficiency of oxygen can cause cyanosis. The fingers go blue, swell up and become extremely painful. As the attack passes, the pain becomes unbearable, involving a sensation of throbbing and of needles pricking at the ends of the fingers; then circulation returns and the hand looks normal again.

Generally speaking, these symptoms represent a relatively minor problem; but they can also accompany diabetes, pressure on a nerve, cervical arthritis or periarthritis in the shoulder, a blood disorder or a neurological disorder.

/ *Exercises for relief*

1   Improving the blood supply to the autonomic nervous pathways of the arms

These pathways start in the neck before crossing the shoulder and descending into the arm.

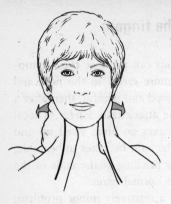

To operate on the autonomic nervous pathways of the neck

Place the palms of your hands on the side of your neck, at the lowest point.
● apply pressure to both sides of your neck in a backwards direction; exhale
● maintain the pressure and breathe shallowly
● relax; inhale
● repeat the procedure 10 times.

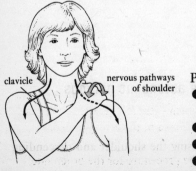

clavicle

nervous pathways
of shoulder

Put the palm of your right hand in the depression above your left clavicle.
● apply pressure to the depression against the trapezius muscle behind it; exhale
● maintain the pressure, breathing shallowly
● relax; inhale
● after a series of 10 movements, reverse the procedure for the other side.

The nervous pathways in the arm

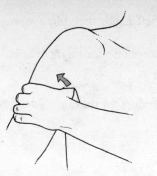

Encircle your arm beneath your right armpit with your left hand. With your left thumb seek the pulse of the axillary artery, around which there is a whole cluster of nerves.

- with your left thumb apply pressure to the arterial pulse point; exhale; feel an 'electric current' sensation pass down your arm
- relax; inhale
- after a series of 10 applications, reverse the procedure for the other side.

With your left hand, encircle your right arm half-way down. Let your left thumb seek the pulse of the brachial artery, around which there is a cluster of nerves.

- apply pressure with your left thumb on the area of the artery; exhale
- relax; inhale
- after a series of 10 applications, reverse the procedure for the other side.

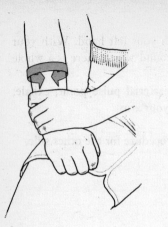

Sit down and encircle your right wrist with your left hand, then place your hands on your left or right thigh.
- apply pressure to your right wrist by pressing down on your thigh; exhale
- maintain the pressure and breathe shallowly
- relax; inhale
- after a series of 10 applications, reverse the procedure for the other side.

2   To improve the working of the muscles

Stretch out your right arm horizontally at a slight angle to the rear, and close your fist.
- turn your closed fist around the axis of your arm in a backwards direction; inhale
- turn your fist in the opposite direction around the axis of your arm; exhale

- after a series of 10 exercises, reverse the procedure for the other side.

3 To improve respiration

Sit down with your hands clasping your opposite elbows.
- rise up from the seat, drawing up your chest with the help of the muscles in the front of your neck; inhale
- relax; exhale
- repeat the exercise 10 times.

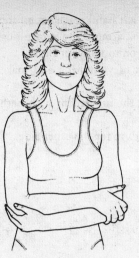

// *Strengthening exercises*

1 Loosening up the back of the neck and the shoulders

Place your hands with the fingers interlocked, over the back of your neck, keeping your arms relaxed.
- apply pressure to the muscles at the back of your neck by bringing the palms of your hands together; exhale
- maintain the pressure and breathe shallowly
- relax the pressure; inhale
- repeat the procedure 10 times.

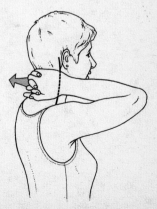

Put your head in the neutral position, then with your left hand reach round the back of your neck and let your first three fingers hook around the protruding part of the top of the spine. Place your right hand flat on top of your head.

● lower your left elbow so as to stretch the back of your neck and make your head turn to the right; exhale

● let your head spring back lightly, accompanying the movement with both hands; inhale

● after a series of 10 movements, reverse the procedure for the other side.

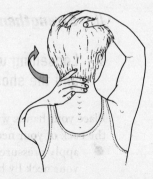

For other exercises see *Cervical spondylosis*, pp. 69–85, and *Tension in the back of the neck and in the shoulders*, pp. 79–85.

2 Working the arm muscles

Get on all fours and stretch your arms and legs while maintaining a stable posture, with the weight of your body evenly distributed.

● lift up your head and lower your pelvis so that
  you take your body weight on to your
  arms; exhale
● return to the starting position; inhale
● repeat the exercise 10 times.

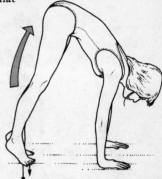

Put your hands behind your body so that they are resting on a chair or another low piece of furniture, and bend your legs to distribute your body weight.

● push on your hands so that you stretch them, with the help of a push from your feet, if necessary; inhale
● return to the starting position; exhale
● repeat the exercise 10 times.

3   Respiration

Lie on the ground, and using your elbows on the ground and your hands around the bottom of your back, raise your pelvis; stretch out your legs, making sure that the back of your neck is not under excessive pressure.

- breathe normally in this position for a few moments; then exhale but do not breathe in yet
- when you feel the need for air, bring your pelvis to the ground while inhaling
- continue to inhale as you stretch the whole of your body out on the ground
- repeat the exercise 10 times.

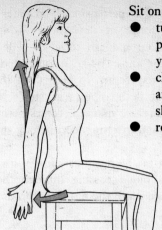

Sit on a chair with your arms hanging loosely on either side.
- turn the palms of your hands outwards, pushing backwards a little to straighten your back; inhale
- close your hands, turning the fists inwards and bringing your arms forwards slightly so that your back curves; exhale
- repeat the exercise 10 times.

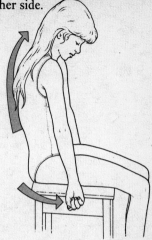

Haemorrhoids

Haemorrhoids are a common ailment – one in four of us suffers from them. Even though there is, of course, nothing to be ashamed of, we can be perplexed and embarrassed about them.

A sedentary life, obesity and constipation are the most frequent causes of haemorrhoids, though they can also result from pregnancy, a tumour in the pelvic region, a heart problem or portal hypertension. Too much rich food (game, highly spiced dishes, various forms of alcohol) or sitting for long periods – all too frequent a habit in our modern society – will produce a feeling of heaviness and burning in the anus. When passing stools we may notice a little blood, then everything may return to normal. If the problem persists, however, a small swelling of flesh appears as stools are passed. Eventually this prolapse (a descent of organic tissue) becomes permanent and is sometimes accompanied by intense pain, irritating local itching and frequent bleeding.

Haemorrhoids are due to a dilation of the haemorrhoidal veins after they have become congested. The venous blood passing through the liver, or returning up the legs, finds it difficult to reach the heart and produces varices in the end section of the digestive tract.

Venous circulation can be improved by:
● rhythmical contraction of the leg muscles
● respiration, especially inhalation, which induces the suction of venous blood towards the heart
● the autonomic nervous system, which produces contraction of the muscular fibres of the vein walls
● steady walking or running, which produces an impact on the veins in the soles of the feet
● drainage of a congested liver
● improved bowel function.

I   Exercises for relief

1   To improve the blood supply to the nervous centres and pathways at the bottom of the back and in the sacrum

These govern the physiological process which enables stools to be passed.

Lie on the floor some distance from a wall, so that your legs are slightly bent and your feet rest on the wall; let your arms lie relaxed on the ground.
- push both feet against the wall; inhale; feel the pressure at the bottom of your back, and increase or decrease your pushing to direct the pressure on to your loins and pelvis
- maintain the pressure, breathing shallowly
- relax the pressure without moving your feet on the wall; exhale
- repeat the exercise 10 times.

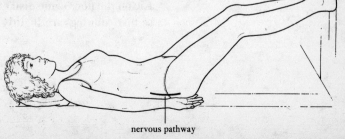

nervous pathway

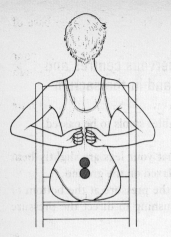

Sit on a chair, with both fists against your lumbar area below your lower ribs and between your back and the chair-back.

● lean slightly to the rear to squeeze the lumbar area with your fists; inhale
● maintain the pressure and breathe shallowly
● gently come forwards again to release the pressure; exhale
● repeat the exercise 10 times
● operate in the same way all along your lumbar area, then with a hand on the bony protrusion of your sacrum.

2   To restore tone to the muscles of the abdomen and the lumbar area

This reduces the feeling of heaviness and excess pressure in the abdomen.

Lie on the floor some distance from a wall,
so that your legs are slightly bent

and your feet rest on the wall; place the fingers of both hands at the base of your abdomen just above your pubic bone.

● lightly inflate your lungs and simultaneously press down on to your abdomen and upwards towards your head with your fingers (as though you wanted to move your abdomen upwards)

● remain a few moments with the pressure directed upwards towards your head, breathing shallowly

● gradually release the pressure; exhale

● repeat the procedure 10 times, applying pressure all over your lower abdomen.

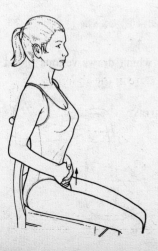

Sit on a chair and place the palms of your hands flat on your lower abdomen, with your fingers touching and your back well braced against the back of the chair.

● inflate your lungs by using the muscles in the front of your neck; draw in your chin and compress your abdomen, applying pressure upwards; inhale

● maintain the pressure and breathe shallowly

● relax the pressure; exhale

● repeat the procedure 10 times over the whole of your lower abdomen.

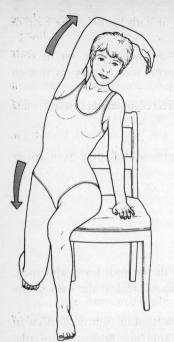

Sit on the side edge of a chair so that your left buttock rests on the chair and the right one is off it. Place your left hand on the chair to maintain your balance, and bring your right arm across over your head.

● simultaneously (a) stretch your right arm to the left and (b) let your right buttock descend; inhale – feel the whole of your right side stretching
● bring your right buttock back up and your right arm back to the right at the same time; exhale
● after a series of 10 movements, reverse the procedure for the other side.

3 To improve respiration

These special exercises to improve the inhalation which draws venous blood towards the heart are most effective.

Put your feet against a wall or on a chair and your arms along the sides of your body.

- slide your arms back along the ground in a circular movement to meet above your head with your fingers entwined, and at the same time inhale slowly
- continue to inhale while stretching the upper part of your body; feel your back arching and your abdomen hollowing
- very gently bend your arms and bring them down in front of your chest with your hands still joined together; exhale normally, without any forcing, so as not to increase the internal abdominal pressure
- unfasten your fingers, slide your arms to the ground, and repeat the exercise 10 times.

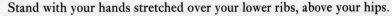

Stand with your hands stretched over your lower ribs, above your hips.
- apply gentle pressure, taking care not to damage your ribs; exhale slowly and fully
- refrain from breathing in for as long as possible – but without forcing
- release the pressure; inhale slowly and deeply
- hold your breath for a few moments
- repeat the exercise 10 times.

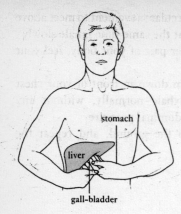

stomach

liver

gall-bladder

4   To help decongest the liver

We should try to eliminate liver congestion, which blocks the venous circulation returning to the heart (the portal venous system).

Sit down, and lean slightly forwards with your fingers hooked under the edge of your right ribs.

● apply pressure and increase it steadily, penetrating underneath your ribs; exhale
● maintain the pressure; breathe shallowly
● release the pressure gradually by drawing your fingers out from under your ribs; inhale
● repeat the movement 10 times
● work in the same way under your left ribs by reversing your hands (this area is often tense, as though in sympathy with the area on the right).

Lie on the ground, and raise your pelvis with the help of your elbows and hands; leave your legs relaxed and bent and your neck free from any excessive pressure.

● exhale, and feel your stomach being pressed against your rib cage; lower your feet towards the ground

- inhale calmly, and feel your feet coming away from the ground
- repeat the exercise 10 times.

// *Strengthening exercises*

Between bouts of pain, our main concern should be to improve the passage of material through the intestines to avoid constipation.

1   To reduce constipation

Sit down with your legs together and place your hands around your knees.
- bring your knees up to your chest; exhale
- push your knees down again until your arms are fully extended; inhale
- repeat the exercise 10 times.

Lie on your back and hook your fingers together above your head; bend your legs and rock them towards your right side.

● turn your head to the left, and at the same time (a) stretch your arms up above your head, and (b) stretch your thighs by pushing down on your knees (if necessary, use your feet to help by pushing them down on the floor); inhale slowly and deeply while doing this

● return to the starting position and relax; exhale

● after a series of 10 movements, reverse the procedure for the other side.

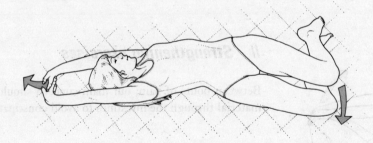

For other exercises see *Constipation*, pp. 223–39.

2   To improve circulation in the legs

Stoop down with your hands on the floor and your arms stretched.
● push down on your feet and stretch your arms, keeping your hands on the floor; inhale deeply
● bring your buttocks down to your heels; exhale
● repeat the exercise 10 times.

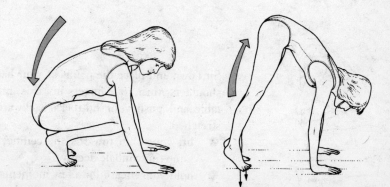

For other exercises see *Heaviness in the legs, varicose veins*, pp. 167–76.

3   To improve respiration

Lie face down on the ground, with your arms bent on either side of your head and your chin on the ground.

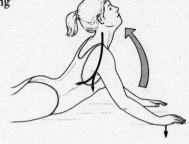

- raise your chin off the ground by pushing on your hands and arching your body backwards; inhale deeply
- relax and return to the floor; exhale
- repeat the exercise 10 times.

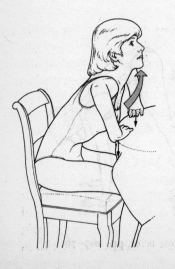

Sit down and place the palms of your hands on a table or desk, level with your shoulders; turn your fingers inwards, raise your elbows, put your chin on the table and push your buttocks backwards on the chair so that your back is stretched.

- lift your chin towards the ceiling, pushing down on your hands at the same time; inhale deeply
- hold your breath for a few moments
- bring your chin down on to the desk, bending your arms; exhale calmly
- repeat the exercise 10 times.

PROBLEMS WITH ARTERIAL TENSION (BLOOD-PRESSURE)

Arterial hypertension (high blood-pressure)

We all suffer from hypertension, but fortunately only occasionally. We should make sure that we know how to take care of ourselves, however, so that we can avoid, later on, being numbered among the 15 per cent or more of the population who suffer from chronic high blood-pressure (usually diagnosed as blood-pressure over 140/90 mm of mercury). In the course of a day things go wrong, we have moments of joy, worry, hate, physical effort, and we eat large meals. All these factors can make our blood-pressure fluctuate and cause it to rise.

Every time the heart contracts, the pumping of blood as it flows through the body causes an increase in pressure on the artery walls. Each time the heart refills, this pressure decreases. The danger with hypertension is that this incessant bombardment of the arteries causes their gradual deterioration, and eventually serious damage occurs, with the possibility that arteries in the brain may ultimately be affected. The nerve cells, which are deprived of oxygen in the event of a stroke, die after three minutes of such deprivation – and they cannot be renewed. A stroke brings the risk of paralysis, speech problems, blindness, heart and respiratory disorders, deep coma and even death; not to mention its direct effects on the heart, aorta or kidneys.

While in 50 per cent of cases of hypertension the cause stems from kidney damage, in the other 50 per cent no organic cause is detectable. High blood-pressure has been called 'directors' disease', 'managers' stress', etc., in other words it affects, in particular, people who drive themselves too hard and are quick to get worked up and irritated. Also affected are those who are fond of tobacco, coffee, alcohol, and who like to eat well – generally with a tendency to obesity. Their poor muscular tone corresponds with their lack of enthusiasm for physical exercise.

Hypertension usually manifests itself through small signs, such as headaches, ringing in the ears, and a frequent desire to urinate in the night; but quite often the only obvious abnormality is a raised blood-pressure reading. Whatever the cause (detectable or undetectable), this disorder is characterized by a permanent state of spasm in the small arteries and a forced reduction in blood space. In other words, as the blood-pressure rises, a given volume of blood will have the capacity of its reservoir reduced. As a result, there is a risk of the arterial walls rupturing, with consequent adverse effects on the blood supply to the cells.

As we all know, most people who lead a sedentary life do not look after their legs too well. Just moving from a chair to a car does not give them a chance to mobilize their large muscle masses to pump a significant volume of blood through their arteries. The simplest exercise – such as walking at a fast pace or jogging – opens the arteries and does them good. It enables the body to call upon a supplementary reservoir of blood flowing through the legs, which because of its low location can help to diminish the high blood-pressure found higher up the body quite naturally. A case of the legs coming to the aid of the head!

/ *Exercises for relief*

1   To activate the circulation in the legs

Walking is the simplest way to achieve this. In addition we could practise the following exercises.

Stand up beside a table or other piece of furniture, and place your left hand on it.
- lower yourself on to your heels by bending your knees; exhale
- stand up straight, with the help of your left hand, without leaning forward; inhale
- repeat the exercise 10 times.

In this way we stimulate, in particular, our thigh muscles.

Lie down with your knees bent and your right leg over your left leg; put your hands on your knees.

- pull both knees in towards you; exhale; feel your right thigh muscles stretching
- relax; inhale
- after a series of 10 movements, reverse the procedure for the other side.

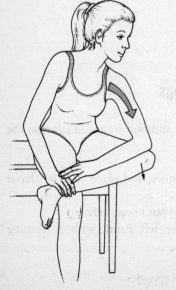

Sit down, put your left foot on your right knee, and place your hands on your left leg.

- bend the top of your body towards your left knee; exhale, feeling the stretching at the back of your left thigh
- relax; inhale
- after a series of 10 movements, reverse the procedure for the other side.

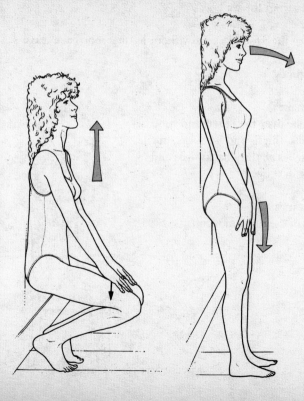

To exercise the whole of the body

Crouch down with your back against a wall and your hands on your knees, and look straight ahead.

- push on your knees and stand up, sliding your back up the wall; inhale
- stand up straight with your hands on the front of your thighs, and look straight ahead
- slowly slide your hands down your thighs to your knees or a little lower; exhale, feeling the back of both your legs stretching
- now lean forward with your hands on the front of your legs
- lift up your head and flatten your back; inhale
- slide your buttocks down the wall and return to the starting position; exhale
- repeat the exercise 10 times.

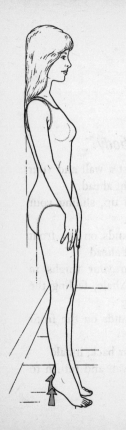

Stand with your back against a wall (for greater stability) and your feet slightly apart, about 8 inches from the wall.

● rise up on tip-toe; inhale
● bring your feet down to the ground again without letting your back leave the wall; exhale
● repeat the exercise 10 times.

Sit down on the edge of a chair.

● stretch your legs out, one over the other, and squeeze together your feet, knees, thighs and buttocks; inhale, so that your body stretches slightly backwards and increases the breathing in action
● relax; exhale
● repeat the exercise 10 times
● reverse legs and perform the same movements.

2   Improving digestion

By assisting digestion we avoid an accumulation of blood in the centre of the body. This can improve peripheral blood flow: something we should aim for in cases of arterial hypertension. See *Digestive pains in the abdomen*, pp. 216–50.

3   Diminishing the discharge of adrenaline, which causes high blood-pressure

The suprarenal glands, situated above the kidneys, are responsible for the discharge of the hormones adrenaline and noradrenaline. These substances are capable of causing spasms in the arteries and a rise in blood-pressure. Exercises can improve the blood supply to the nervous pathways of the back.

Sit on a chair; put your fists on each side of your spine, level with your lower ribs, and place your back against the back of the chair so that your fists are squeezed between your back and the chair-back.

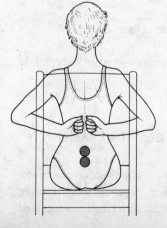

● let the top of your body go backwards; inhale, and feel the pressure of your fists on your back
● maintain the pressure and breathe shallowly
● let the top of your body come slightly forwards again; exhale
● repeat the movements 10 times.

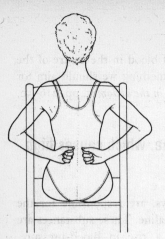

// *Strengthening exercises*

1   To improve the blood supply to the kidneys

By improving the circulation in the area of the kidneys, we can help them to eliminate urine more effectively.

Wedge your fists between your back and the back of a chair, just beneath your lower ribs, on either side of your spine.
- lean back; inhale, and feel your lower back being squeezed by your fists
- maintain the pressure and breathe shallowly
- let your upper body come gently forwards again; exhale
- repeat the movements 10 times
- repeat along your lower back (two different positions for your fists should be sufficient).

2   To encourage the elimination of urine from the bladder

Just as tapping the lower abdominal region in front of the bladder causes the reflex passage of urine, so a series of alternating pressing and relaxing movements acts in the same way. Stimulation of the sacrum (the bone situated

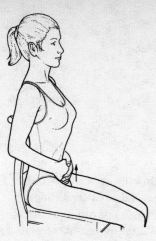

at the base of the spine) will, by activation of the autonomic nervous pathways issuing at this point, also result in the passing of urine.

Place the fingers of one hand over those of the other, just above your pubic bone.
- inflate your lungs and pull in your abdomen, pressing inwards with the help of your fingers; inhale
- maintain the pressure and breathe shallowly
- relax the pressure; exhale
- repeat the procedure 10 times.

This exercise can be practised upright or lying down.

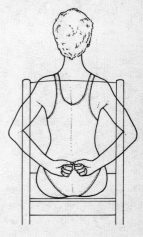

Wedge your fists between your back and the back of a chair, level with the sacrum, between your hip bones, just beneath the lumbar vertebrae.
- lean slightly backwards; inhale, and feel your sacrum being squeezed by your fists
- maintain the pressure, breathing shallowly
- let your trunk come forward again; exhale
- repeat the movements 10 times.

3   Exercising the legs, see *Exercises for relief*, pp. 199–200.

4 Reducing obesity

Many people need to lose weight. See *Obesity*, pp. 338–47.

5 Reducing stress, see *Stress*, pp. 258–69.

Orthostatic arterial hypotension

We may sometimes feel giddy, dazed or generally unwell; or feel our heart racing when we get out of bed suddenly or when we stand up after sitting or crouching for a long time. We can also experience the same symptoms after standing for a long time in an overheated or stressful atmosphere. We are all potential victims of hypotension (low blood-pressure).

Hypotension is usually diagnosed when blood-pressure falls below 100/55 mm of mercury. This results in the cells of the body receiving insufficient nourishment. Hypotension may be due to specific organic causes: neurological or endocrine disease, diabetes, a serious infection, anaemia, convalescence from an illness or a digestive malfunction leading to undernourishment. It can also be caused by medication taken for hypertension, or by insomnia.

The body's reactions to a bout of hypotension are salutary: they compel us to lie down – a position favourable to a horizontal blood flow, which does not have to adapt to body weight.

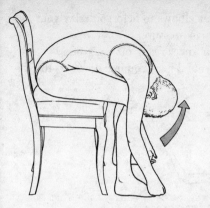

I Exercises for relief

1   To improve the blood supply to the brain

The body always gives priority to the blood supply of the brain and heart in cases of hypotension, so let's help it.

Lean forward, with your upper body resting on your thighs, your head between your legs, and your arms hanging relaxed by your sides.
- inhale while raising your chin slightly
- exhale while letting your head drop down again
- repeat the movements 10 times.

Kneel down and put your forehead on the ground, or turn your head to one side on the ground with your arms relaxed along each side of your body.
- inflate your chest; inhale
- deflate your chest; exhale
- repeat the movements 10 times.

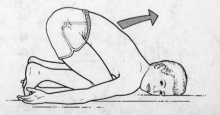

Lie on the ground and lift your pelvis; use your elbows to help you relax your legs, making sure your neck is not under excessive pressure.
- inflate your abdomen; inhale, and feel your knees rising off the ground
- deflate your abdomen; exhale, and feel your knees coming down to the ground
- repeat the exercise 10 times.

This exercise promotes a considerable flow of blood to the head.

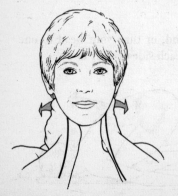

Place the palms of your hands over the sides of your neck.
- apply pressure towards the rear on both sides of your neck
- maintain the pressure and breathe shallowly
- relax the pressure; inhale
- repeat the procedure 10 times.

You will immediately feel a flow of blood to your face and head. This exercise treats the autonomic nervous pathways in the neck.

2 To improve oxygen supply

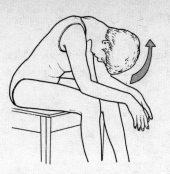

Nerve cells are very sensitive to a lowering of their oxygen supply, so we should try to remedy this deficiency.

Place your elbows on your knees, let your head hang down, and relax your arms and hands.
- lift your chin and head towards the rear; inhale slowly
- return to a relaxed position, with your head hanging; exhale
- repeat the movements 10 times.

Sit on your toes with your knees together, your forehead on the ground, your arms relaxed and half bent and the palms of your hands on the ground.
- push on your hands, stretch your arms and lift your chin towards the ceiling; inhale deeply
- bring your forehead back to the ground, bending your arms; exhale
- repeat the exercise 10 times.

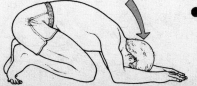

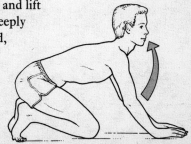

3 To calm spasms in the digestive tract

An application of slow, prolonged pressure will help to relieve tensions which are often due to overwork. Lying down on your stomach is the best position for this.

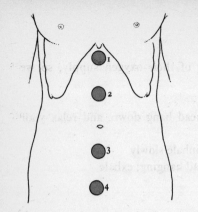

1 solar plexus
2 upper intestinal plexus
3 lower intestinal plexus
4 plexus of the lower abdomen

Pressure to the solar plexus

Place your fingers under your sternum.
- increase the pressure steadily; exhale
- maintain the pressure and breathe shallowly
- steadily and slowly reduce the pressure; inhale
- repeat the procedure 10 times
- repeat the procedure with the other plexuses.

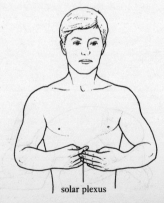

solar plexus

Pressure to the areas below the ribs

Hook your fingers under your right ribs.

- increase the pressure steadily and slowly, penetrating under your ribs with your fingers; exhale
- maintain the pressure and breathe shallowly
- reduce the pressure slowly, withdrawing your fingers from beneath your ribs; inhale
- repeat the procedure 10 times
- repeat the procedure under your left ribs.

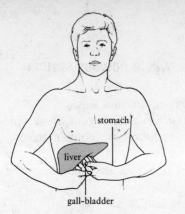

To help the functioning of the large intestine

Place your fingers over your right groin.

- apply pressure slowly; exhale
- maintain the pressure and breathe shallowly
- relax the pressure; inhale
- repeat along the length of your colon at the points indicated in the illustration.

// *Strengthening exercises*

1 To improve the blood supply to the whole nervous system

Lie with your buttocks against a wall and your hands on your knees.
- simultaneously push on the wall with your feet and on your knees with your hands so as to raise your body gradually off the ground, starting with your lumbar area; inhale
- stop for a few moments at each section of your back and spine, lingering on any more tender areas
- gently relax the pressure on your hands and feet; exhale
- bring your buttocks down to the ground; exhale
- repeat the procedure several times.

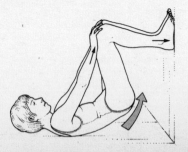

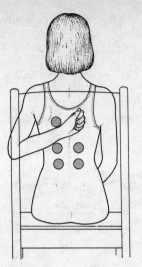

Sit on a chair and place your left fist on the ridge of muscle to the right of your spine so that it is wedged between your back and the back of the chair.

- lean backwards so that you apply pressure to your back; inhale
- maintain the pressure and breathe shallowly
- come gently forwards again; exhale
- repeat the movements 10 times
- operate along the whole of your back as indicated
- change fists to operate along the other side.

2 The muscles at the back of the neck and in the back

By strengthening these muscles we help the body to maintain a better posture when standing up.

Lie on the ground on your front, with your arms relaxed beside your head and your chin on the ground.

- lift up your chin and push down on your hands without arching your back too much; exhale
- lower your body to the ground; inhale
- repeat the exercise at a fairly steady rhythm, then rest for a few moments on the ground.

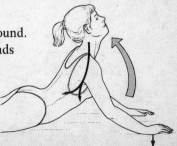

Lie on your front with your arms stretched in front of your head; turn your head to the right, and bend your left leg.
- accentuate the stretching of your left arm; inhale
- relax; exhale
- accentuate the stretching of your right leg; inhale
- relax; exhale
- accentuate the simultaneous stretching of your left arm and your right leg; inhale
- relax; exhale

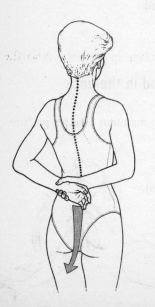

- after a series of 10 movements, reverse the procedure for the other side.

Stand up with your hands behind your back, and let your right hand take hold of your left wrist.
- stretch your arms by pulling your left wrist downwards as far as possible – this will straighten up your back and bring the back of your neck towards the rear; inhale
- relax; exhale
- after a series of 10 movements, reverse the procedure for the other side.

3   Treatment of the suprarenal glands

Sit on a chair and put your fists behind your back, on either side of your spine, level with your lower ribs. Wedge your fists between your back and the back of the chair.

- lean your trunk backwards; inhale, feeling your back being pressed for a few moments, then breathe shallowly
- let your trunk return forwards; exhale
- repeat the movements 10 times.

Make sure that you apply pressure for a relatively long interval and relax the pressure for a relatively short interval.

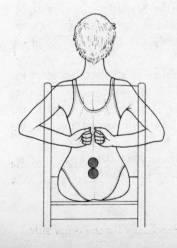

DIGESTIVE PAINS IN THE ABDOMEN

'Liver attack'

Mornings after living it up are really no fun. They usually involve pain under the right ribs with corresponding pain under the shoulder-blade; a tight feeling when you take a deep breath; nausea; vomiting; or a migraine. There may also be premenstrual-type symptoms, or simply a feeling of being out of sorts and irritable.

In fact, a 'liver attack' is not really a liver problem at all. It is an upset in the functioning of the gall-bladder, a small bag on the under-surface of the liver which receives the bile secreted by the liver. Any blockage or spasm in the duct which runs from the gall-bladder to the intestine, carrying bile to help digest fat, can cause these unpleasant symptoms.

Here, as at every stage of the digestive process, we should be aware of the considerable influence exercised by the autonomic nervous system.

I *Exercises for relief*

1 To calm the digestion

The first aim is to reduce any spasmodic activity around the gall-bladder, the solar plexus or in the large intestine. Then we can move on to soothe any pains in the back, which represent trouble in the autonomic nervous pathways controlling the digestion.

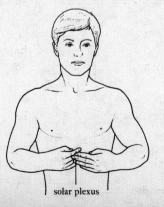

solar plexus

To apply pressure to the solar plexus

Place the closed fingers of one hand on those of the other, and position them at the top of your abdomen, under the point of the sternum.

- apply pressure and increase it steadily; exhale
- maintain constant pressure for a few moments and then breathe shallowly
- release the pressure gradually; inhale
- repeat the procedure 10 times
- repeat on the upper intestinal plexus.

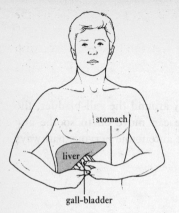

gall-bladder

Applying pressure to the region beneath the right ribs (liver and gall-bladder)

Hook your fingers under your right ribs.
● apply pressure and increase it steadily, penetrating under your ribs, but do not go beyond the point where it becomes painful; exhale
● pause, maintaining steady pressure, then breathe shallowly
● release the pressure gradually; inhale; remove your fingers from under your ribs
● after a series of 10 applications, reverse the procedure for the other side.

Wedge your left hand between your back and the back of a chair, level with your shoulder-blades.
● let your trunk lean backwards, or press firmly against the chair-back: inhale, and feel the pressure from your hand on your back
● maintain the pressure and breathe shallowly
● relax the pressure by bringing your trunk slightly forwards; exhale
● after a series of 10 movements, reverse the procedure for the other side.

VARIATION: You can use your fist to apply more pressure.

autonomic nervous pathways

Lie on the floor with your buttocks against a wall, your feet resting on the wall, and your hands on your knees.

- simultaneously push on the wall with your feet and on your knees with your hands so that you raise your body off the ground gradually, starting with your pelvis; inhale
- pause for a few moments on the tender area of your shoulder-blades and breathe shallowly
- bring your buttocks to the ground, relaxing the pressure; exhale
- repeat the exercise 10 times.

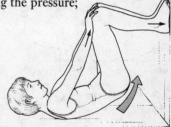

2 Improving respiration

Your breathing may seize up when you inhale deeply, tightening your abdomen and causing spasms. The treatment for this consists of slow, progressive stretching of the whole of the right side of your body. This helps the diaphragm to work better, eases breathing, improves the return of venous blood from the liver to the heart, and reduces pressure on the gall-bladder.

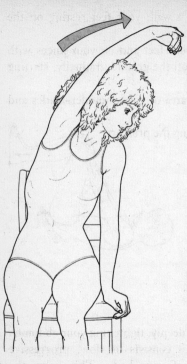

Sit down with your right arm above your head, and place your left arm on the edge of the seat.

● increasingly stretch your right side slowly to the left; inhale
● relax; exhale
● steadily increase the stretching, but do not go beyond a point where it becomes painful
● when you reach the limit of your stretching, inhale as deeply as possible and hold your breath for a few moments
● repeat the exercise several times; then reverse the procedure for the other side.

Half lie on your knees, with your right leg folded under your right side (liver and gall-bladder), your left leg stretched out along the ground, your forehead on the ground, and your arms stretched and relaxed in front of you.

● swell out your abdomen and feel it pressing against your thigh; inhale
● relax your abdomen; exhale
● after a series of 10 movements, reverse the procedure for the other side.

// *Strengthening exercises*

1 Respiration

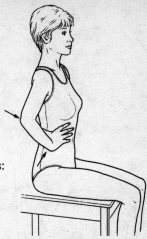

Place your hands on your lower ribs on each side.
- carefully squeeze your ribs; exhale
- maintain the pressure and breathe shallowly
- repeat the procedure 10 times.

The above exercise can also be performed as follows:
- lean forwards as you squeeze
- straighten up as you relax the pressure.

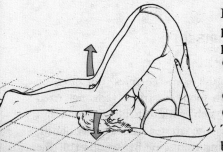

Lie on your back and with the help of your elbows and hands, raise your pelvis off the ground and relax your legs; make sure there is not excessive pressure on the back of your neck.
- inhale slowly and deeply, and feel your hips rocking gently towards the ground
- exhale slowly and fully, and feel your feet coming down to the ground
- repeat the exercise 10 times.

The position of the body in this exercise favours both the drainage of the gallbladder and the working of the respiratory system.

2   The abdominal muscles

Lie on your back with your hands gripping your knees and your legs relaxed and bent.

- bring your knees to your chest with the help of your hands; exhale
- push your knees back again as far as possible; inhale
- repeat the exercise 10 times.

When this exercise becomes easy, practise
it with your hands under your thighs.

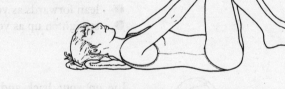

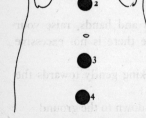

1   solar plexus
2   upper intestinal plexus
3   lower intestinal plexus
4   plexus of the lower abdomen

Gastritis (inflammation of the stomach)

At the root of a variety of digestive upsets the same 'enemies' can often be found: alcohol, tobacco, spices and over-rich food. Gastritis is characterized by a burning sensation in the pit of the stomach, with difficult digestion and sometimes unbearable pain. In addition to the abuses already mentioned, gastritis is often caused by repeatedly rushing meals, or by an upset of the autonomic nervous system. Before you start worrying about whether you have an ulcer or cancer, start by correcting the functioning of the nervous system which governs your digestion.

/ *Exercises for relief*

1 To calm the digestion

This exercise calms the autonomic nervous pathways going to the stomach: if their work of stimulating and inhibiting digestion becomes disordered, gastritis is bound to follow.

To apply pressure to the solar plexus

Put your hands together with the fingers of one hand over the fingers of the other, and position them at the top of your abdomen, under the point of your sternum.

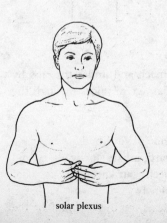

solar plexus

- increase the pressure gradually; exhale
- maintain the pressure for a few moments and breathe shallowly
- gradually relax the pressure; inhale
- repeat the procedure 10 times
- repeat the procedure with your fingers hooked under your left ribs (stomach) then under your right ribs (liver and gall-bladder).

2   Helping the passage of food through the intestines

Apply the same treatment to the other abdominal plexuses, as shown in the illustration. Repeat the alternating pressure-on/pressure-off operation all along the digestive tract, at the points indicated, or on any other area which is tender or painful.

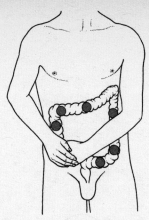

3   Improving respiration

Reduce a feeling of tightness in the pit of the stomach and under the ribs by means of breathing exercises, which improve the passage of juices through the stomach, intestines and gall-bladder.

Place your hands just over the lower ribs, on each side of your body.
* very carefully squeeze your ribs and lean forward; inhale slowly
* pause for a few moments with your head between your knees
* relax the pressure and come up again; inhale slowly
* repeat the exercise 10 times.

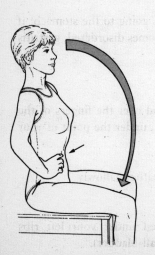

// *Strengthening exercises*

1   To relax the pit of the stomach and under the ribs

Go down on all fours with one knee on the ground, the other bent against
your chest and your head hanging down.
- bend your body more towards your abdomen; exhale
- straighten out your body again by bringing your head up and
  stretching the bent leg backwards and upwards; inhale
- after a series of 10 movements, reverse the procedure
  for the other side.

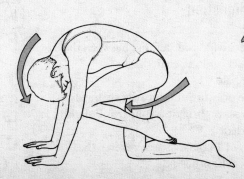

Put your left elbow on your left knee and your right arm above your head.

- extend your right arm, stretching the whole of the right side of your body and your rib cage; inhale
- relax gently; exhale
- after a series of 10 movements, reverse the procedure for the other side.

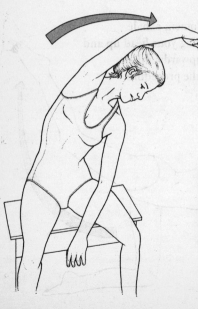

2 Improving the blood supply to the nervous pathways in the back linked with the digestion

Sit on a chair and wedge your left fist between the middle of your back and the chair-back.

- lean back; inhale
- maintain the pressure and breathe shallowly
- relax the pressure, bringing your trunk slightly forwards; exhale
- after a series of 10 movements, reverse the procedure for the other side.

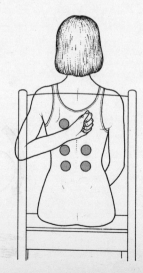

Lie on your back on the ground with your buttocks against a wall, your feet resting on the wall, and your hands on your knees.

- at the same time, push on the wall and on your knees to lift your body gradually off the floor, starting with your hips; inhale
- rest on the middle of your back for a few moments and breathe shallowly
- bring your buttocks down to the ground; exhale
- repeat the exercise several times.

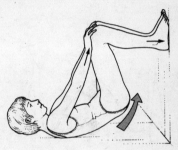

Diarrhoea

Diarrhoea is often accompanied by pain in the intestines (colic). Food poisoning or a variety of other causes – a chill, emotional problems, antibiotics or a food allergy – can bring on an acute attack.

Chronic diarrhoea can be caused by a parasite, or by a kidney or heart deficiency; it can also be the result of a malfunction of the stomach, liver, colon or pancreas. This intestinal hypersecretion and the rapid passage of material through the intestines has to be stemmed, to allow the bowels to be emptied in a normal manner.

1 solar plexus
2 upper intestinal plexus
3 lower intestinal plexus
4 plexus of the lower abdomen

/ *Exercises for relief*

1 To calm the nervous centres and pathways in the abdomen

The aim of this exercise is to reduce the disorderly hyperfunctioning of the intestines, by improving the blood supply to the nervous centres controlling digestion, and to the most painful areas. The best position is to lie comfortably on your front, with your fingers placed over each other to treat each plexus in turn. Apply gently increasing pressure until you reach a point of 'pleasant sensitivity', then pause and breathe naturally for a few moments. Release the pressure carefully, to avoid any jerky movement which might cause pain or an increase in spasm.

Pressure to the solar plexus

Place the fingers of one hand over those of the other at the top of your abdomen under the point of the sternum.

- apply pressure slowly; exhale
- pause a few moments while maintaining constant pressure
- relax the pressure gradually, without any kind of jerkiness; inhale slowly
- repeat the procedure on the other plexuses.

The treatment is the same for the areas beneath the ribs, but this time the fingers should be hooked so that they can penetrate under the ribs.

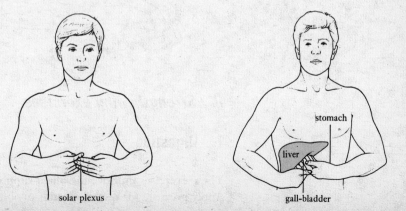

solar plexus

stomach

liver

gall-bladder

2 Respiration

Lie on your back on a bed, with the top of your neck resting on the edge of the bed and your arms hanging backwards and relaxed over the side.
- stretch yourself by lowering your arms a little; inhale, and hold your breath for a few moments
- relax; exhale
- repeat the exercise 10 times.

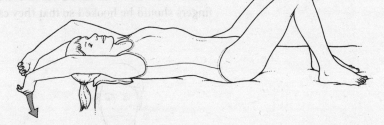

// *Strengthening exercises*

1 Digestion

These exercises improve the blood supply to the autonomic nervous pathways. Apply pressure for several seconds to obtain a calming effect.

Place your buttocks against a wall, with your feet resting on the wall and your hands on your knees.
- push simultaneously against the wall and on your knees so that you lift your body gradually off the ground, starting with your hips; inhale
- maintain this posture for as long as possible without forcing it, and breathe shallowly
- bring your body back to the ground; exhale
- repeat several times.

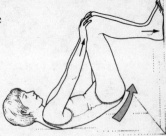

Sit on a chair and place your left fist between the chair-back and a point half-way up your back, on the ridges of muscles to the right of your spinal column.
- lean back so that you squeeze your back; inhale
- maintain the pressure and breathe shallowly
- come forward again to relieve the pressure; exhale
- after a series of 10 movements, reverse the procedure for the other side.

2 Strengthening the respiration

Calm your abdomen by practising large, slow breathing exercises.

Lie on your front, with your arms bent level with your head and your chin on the ground.
- raise up your chin by pushing down on your hands and arching your back inwards; inhale
- hold your breath for a few moments
- relax and come down to the ground again; exhale
- repeat the exercise several times.

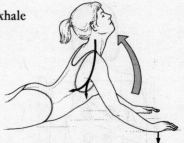

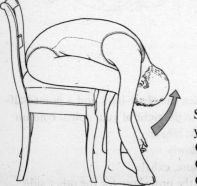

Sit on a chair and bend forward, then put your chest between your thighs, your head between your legs and let your arms hang loosely.
- lift your chin; inhale calmly
- let your head come down again; exhale
- repeat the movements 10 times.

Constipation

The evacuation of the bowels is an automatic function which terminates the digestive process. The muscles of the rectum, when it is full, contract, those of the pelvic floor relax, the sphincters open, and the faeces are eliminated under pressure from the muscles of the abdomen and rectum.

Bad eating habits, insufficient green vegetables, drinking between meals, a sedentary life, lack of exercise – all these can cause this automatic process to be upset. Most of us are very good at mental sport and intellectual exercise, but we move our legs and body very little. With our hectic lives, in which we are always short of time, we forget the primitive reflexes we had when we were small: moving about, running, walking and breathing plenty of fresh air, we were not so likely to be constipated in those days.

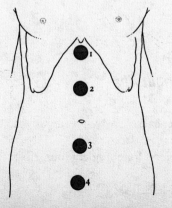

1   solar plexus
2   upper intestinal plexus
3   lower intestinal plexus
4   plexus of the lower abdomen

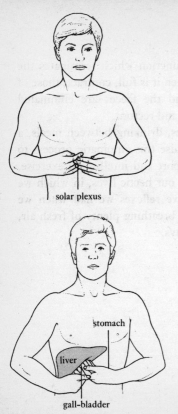

solar plexus

stomach

liver

gall-bladder

/ *Exercises for relief*

1 To act on the nervous centres and pathways of the abdomen

Applying pressure to the solar plexus

Place the fingers of one hand over the fingers of the other, and lay them flat at the top of your abdomen under the point of your sternum.

● apply pressure; exhale
● maintain the pressure and breathe shallowly
● relax the pressure; inhale
● repeat the movements 10 times
● repeat the same movements on all the plexuses.

Applying pressure to the area under the right ribs

Hook your fingers under your right ribs.

● apply pressure, penetrating under your ribs; exhale
● maintain the pressure and shallow breathe
● relax the pressure and withdraw your fingers from under your ribs; inhale
● reverse the procedure for the area under your left ribs.

Applying pressure to the abdomen

Put your fingers together and place them flat above your right groin.

- apply pressure; exhale
- maintain the pressure and breathe shallowly
- relax the pressure; inhale
- repeat the movements 10 times
- repeat the treatment along the path of your colon at the points indicated.

This treatment by intermittent pressure differs from that for diarrhoea, as here it is applied with a quicker rhythm.

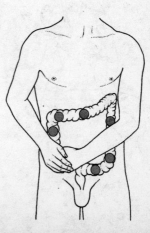

2 To improve respiration

Stimulation of the respiration is vital. (Some people even say that smoking their first cigarette in the morning helps open their bowels!)

Sit down and put your left leg over your right leg, your right hand on your left thigh and your left hand on the edge of your chair.

● push on your left thigh with your right hand; exhale, and feel the rotation of your trunk to the right
● relax; inhale
● after a series of 10 movements, reverse the procedure for the other side.

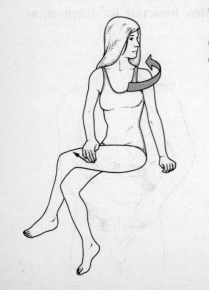

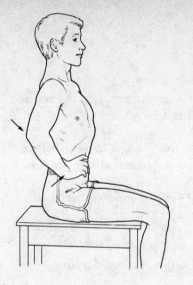

Stimulation of the abdominal muscles

Put your hands on your hips.
- squeeze your hips while exhaling
- maintain the pressure a few moments; breathe shallowly
- relax the pressure while inhaling
- repeat the exercise 10 times.

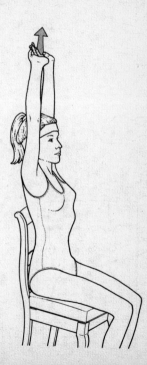

Stimulating the diaphragm

With fingers entwined, put your hands on your head.
- stretch your arms above your head; inhale
- bring your hands down on to your head; exhale
- repeat the exercise 10 times.

// *Strengthening exercises*

1 Evacuation of the bowels

This exercise stimulates the autonomic nervous centres controlling the evacuation of the bowels, in the area of the lower back and the sacrum.

Sit on a chair and place your left fist against your back at a point between your lower ribs and your pelvis, so that your fist is wedged between your back and the chair-back.

- press against the chair-back; inhale, and feel the pressure exercised by your fist on your back
- maintain the pressure and breathe shallowly
- relax the pressure by leaning slightly forwards; exhale
- repeat the treatment down your lower back, then on your sacrum
- reverse the procedure for the other side.

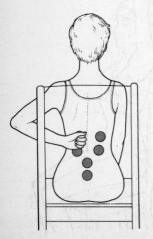

2 Strengthening the respiration

Stimulate the abdomen by practising respiratory exercises at a brisk rhythm.

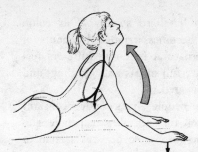

Lie on your front with your arms bent level with your head and your chin on the ground.
- raise your chin by pushing on your hands and arching your back inwards; inhale
- relax and come down to the ground again; exhale
- repeat the exercise 10 times.

Lie down on your back with your hands on your knees and your legs bent.
- bring your knees up to your chest with the help of your hands; exhale
- move your knees away from your chest with your hands; inhale
- perform the exercise at a quick rhythm
- repeat the exercise 10 times.

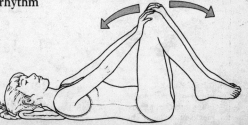

VARIATION: Do the exercise sitting on a chair and leaning against the chair-back.

Spasmodic colitis

This disorder is a product of our so-called 'civilized society'. Our colon complains by way of attacks of colic, and becomes irritated by bouts of diarrhoea or constipation which seem to alternate at random. Sufferers feel that their abdomen is unpleasantly 'puffed up', full of gas and gurgling, and that their bowels have not been completely evacuated.

Spasmodic colitis most frequently attacks people living under constant stress and worry – students before examinations, for example – or people who abuse laxatives. It is a typical example of the autonomic nervous system of the digestive tract being upset by the overwork of its two components, the sympathetic and the parasympathetic nerves: the one working to slow down the passage of food through the intestines, and the other ordering it to accelerate.

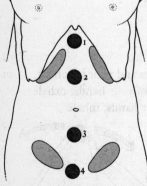

1 solar plexus
2 upper intestinal plexus
3 lower intestinal plexus
4 plexus of the lower abdomen

/ *Exercises for relief*

1   To calm the nervous centres and pathways of the abdomen

First we should treat the inflammation of the colon, as if it were a case of diarrhoea (even if you *are* suffering from constipation). Lying face down is the most effective position.

Start by applying pressure to the plexuses, indicated in the illustration by circles (*opposite*); then apply pressure in the shaded areas as follows.

● apply pressure with both hands placed flat, one on top of the other, increasing the pressure steadily; exhale

● maintain steady pressure for a few moments and breathe shallowly

● relax the pressure gradually to avoid any jerky movements; inhale

● repeat the procedure 10 times.

2   To calm the autonomic nervous pathways in the back

The command centres in contact with the spinal column are hyperactive and produce sensations of heaviness, discomfort or pain which we should try to eliminate. Be careful to carry out the treatment slowly.

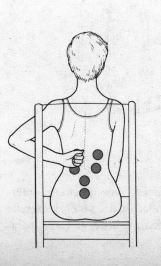

Place your left fist on your back at a point between the lower ribs and the pelvis, so that it is wedged against the back of the chair.

● gradually lean back; inhale, and feel the pressure on your back from your fist

● maintain the steady pressure for a few moments, breathing shallowly

● gradually relax the pressure by leaning slightly forward; exhale

● repeat the treatment over your lower back, then on your sacrum

● reverse the procedure for the other side.

Lie on your back, with your thighs at right angles to your abdomen, your feet resting on the wall, your right hand flat under your lumbar area, and your left arm along your body.

- gently rock your knees to the right without moving your feet; exhale
- pause for a few moments
- bring your knees back to the starting position; inhale
- repeat the exercise, moving your hand down along your lumbar area and on to your sacrum.

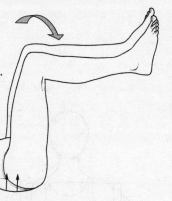

3 To encourage better oxygenation of the body

To restore a balanced digestive system, practise deep, slow breathing, interspersed with prolonged, spontaneous (not controlled) pauses. This exercise helps to regulate the functioning of both the sympathetic and the parasympathetic nervous systems.

Rest the top of your neck on the edge of a bed, with your arms hanging down relaxed over the side.
- stretch the upper part of your body by lowering both arms a little; inhale
- hold your breath for a few moments
- relax your arms, exhale
- repeat the exercise 10 times.

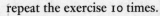

Lie down on the ground and bring both knees up to your chest.
- squeeze your knees against your chest; exhale
- push your knees away and place your feet on a wall or your legs on a chair, while inhaling slowly and deeply from your abdomen
- hold your breath for a few moments
- repeat the exercise 10 times.

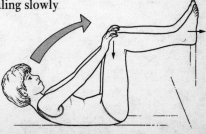

// *Strengthening exercises*

1 To reduce a state of distress and anxiety

This exercise involves pressure on the neck, chest and abdomen. It improves the blood supply to the top half of the back, where the nervous pathways which control the heart, breathing and digestion run.

Lie down, and with the help of your elbows and hands, raise your pelvis off the ground so that your legs remain relaxed and bent and the back of your neck is free from excessive pressure.

- exaggerate the movement by pushing lightly on your lumbar area to lower your legs; exhale
- relax without returning to the ground; inhale
- repeat the action 10 times
- then return to the ground with a long breath in.

For other exercises, see *Stress*, pp. 258–69.

2   To reduce stress

Lie on your back on the floor, with your arms bent under the back of your neck; bend your legs, and put your knees together and feet apart.

- push (a) on the floor with your feet and (b) on your knees in the direction of your feet, to stretch your lower back; inhale
- relax and come down to the ground so that you are back in your starting position; exhale
- repeat the exercise 10 times.

Be careful not to arch your body too much, but rather to stretch your back without moving your arms or head.

For other exercises, see *Stress*, pp. 258–69.

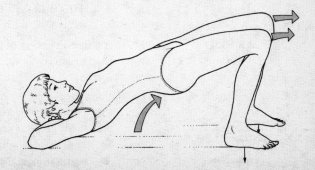

Flatulence

Sometimes an abnormal amount of gas may congest your stomach or your intestines. The distension which follows produces a discomfort in the abdomen that can be quite painful. Digestion becomes difficult and is often punctuated by unpleasant belching.

While flatulence can be an indication of a stomach complaint or of a liver, bladder, or even heart problem, it is also often caused by disorders of the autonomic nervous system as a result of physical or mental overwork.

/ *Exercises for relief*

1   To calm the digestion

A sluggish action of the intestines accompanied by spasms in the digestive tract is characteristic of flatulence, and we should try to calm this disordered activity.

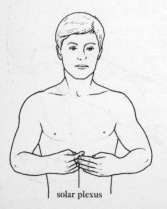

solar plexus

Put your fingers together and place your hands flat at the top of your abdomen, on your solar plexus.
- apply and slowly increase pressure; exhale
- maintain a constant pressure and breathe shallowly

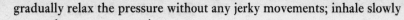

- gradually relax the pressure without any jerky movements; inhale slowly
- repeat the treatment 10 times
- repeat the treatment under your right ribs and under your left ribs, then on the other plexuses of your abdomen.

2 To improve the respiration

Entwine your fingers and put your arms above your head. Stretch the upper part of your body to the right, then to the left, while inhaling slowly.
- relax the stretching; exhale
- repeat the exercise 10 times
- repeat, stretching both arms at the same time.

VARIATION: This exercise can also be performed in a lying position, which is preferable.

// *Strengthening exercises*

1   General exercise for relaxing the abdomen

Stand up with your legs apart and your hands on your hips, and keep the top of your body still.

- make circular movements with your hips; inhale as the hips go forward, exhale as they go back
- repeat the procedure 10 times
- reverse the direction of the movement.

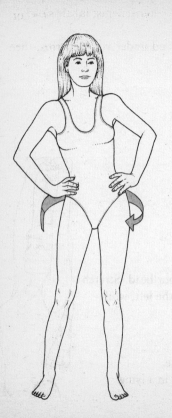

Put your buttocks against a wall, with your feet apart and your legs stretched; then lean forward, letting your head and arms hang down.

- breathe in and out a few times in this position
- swing your arms and head to the right; exhale
- return to the central position; inhale
- swing your arms and head to the left; exhale
- return to the central position; inhale
- repeat the exercise 10 times
- to straighten up, put your hands on your knees and push on your hands.

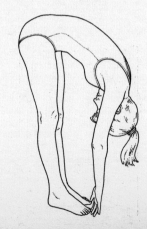

Lie down on the ground, bring your knees up to your chest and put your hands on your knees.

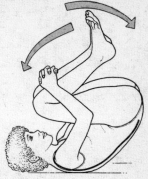

- let yourself roll backwards; exhale
- roll forwards again; inhale
- repeat the exercise 10 times.

2 Treatment of the nervous centres and pathways in the back

Sit on a chair and wedge your left fist between the centre of your back, below your right shoulder-blade, and the chair-back.

- lean back against your fist and the chair-back; inhale
- maintain the pressure and breathe shallowly
- relax the pressure by leaning slightly forward; exhale
- after a series of 10 movements, reverse the procedure for the other side.

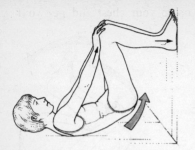

Lie with your buttocks against a wall, then place your feet on the wall with your hands on your knees.

● push on the wall with your feet and on your knees with your hands to raise your body gradually off the ground, starting with your pelvis; inhale
● remain for a few moments on the middle part of your back and breathe shallowly
● bring your buttocks back to the ground; exhale
● repeat the exercise several times.

3 Treatment for respiration

This exercise is to practise breathing which is centred particularly on your abdomen, without any kind of jerking.

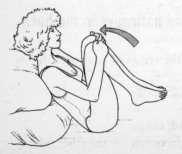

Lie down on the ground with your back preferably raised up, your legs bent, and your hands on your knees.

● bring your knees up smoothly to your chest with your hands; exhale
● push your knees down again with your hands while inhaling calmly
● repeat the exercise 10 times.

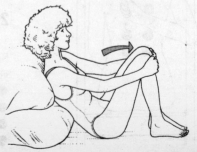

NERVOUS INSTABILITY

Anxiety

Worry, anxiety and distress are the terms we generally use to express escalating degrees of psychological insecurity. This anxiety may take the form of a permanent state of worry without any definable cause. It can occupy our mind completely, and obscure plans for our future and that of those near and dear to us. We feel permanently 'down in the dumps' and cannot rid ourselves of the feeling of imminent catastrophe. This state of mind sometimes relates to a particular situation: some personal conflict, or a serious problem with a relationship. It can eventually lead to depression; but, generally speaking, anxiety depends on our individual reaction to circumstances. Our interpretation of past events is often influenced by our physical or mental state in the present. If we 'get out of bed on the right side' everything seems rosy, but if we 'get out of bed on the wrong side' life looks pretty black. Yet the real world has not changed.

In fact, anxiety, far from being a mental problem, is a physical phenomenon. It often manifests itself as a 'ball' of anxiety lodged tight in our throat, a 'heavy bar' lying on our stomach or a 'tight vice' that stops us breathing. It can make us suffer heart palpitations, pains in the abdomen, headaches and dizziness, an overwhelming desire to pass water or empty our bowels, backache, or sleeping problems.

We all experience this kind of upset at some time in our lives. It's when the symptoms occur again and again that it becomes an illness. These emotional states represent an upset of the autonomic nervous system, and we should work to restore it to health. The most natural remedy is a few nights' really good rest, but we often need the company of friends to help us get over it, and we should certainly consult our doctor.

/ *Exercises for relief*

You will notice that most of the symptoms typical of a bout of anxiety affect the front part of the body: the lump in our throat, the feeling of tightness in our chest, or the knot in our stomach. And it's primarily from here that we operate.

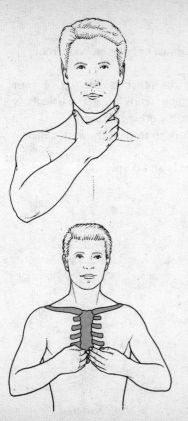

1   To calm local sensations of tightness

In the throat

Lightly grip the front of your throat with your right hand.
● exhale slowly through your mouth, gently squeezing your throat
● maintain the pressure and breathe shallowly
● relax the pressure and inhale slowly and deeply through your mouth
● close your mouth and hold your breath for a few moments
● repeat the procedure 10 times.

In the chest

Place the fingers of both hands on your sternum.
● apply pressure with your fingers, increasing it steadily; exhale slowly
● maintain the pressure and breathe shallowly
● relax the pressure; inhale slowly through your mouth
● repeat the procedure 10 times
● operate in the same way all along your sternum.
VARIATION: Apply pressure with the palms of your hands placed over one another.

In the abdomen

The most effective positions for this are sitting down or lying on your front.

Place the fingers of one hand over those of the other at the top of your abdomen on the solar plexus – an area which tends to get particularly 'knotted' (use the same position of the hands for the other plexuses).

● apply gentle pressure, slowly and deeply enough to calm the area; exhale
● maintain the pressure and breathe shallowly
● gradually relax the pressure and inhale slowly and deeply
● repeat the procedure 10 times.

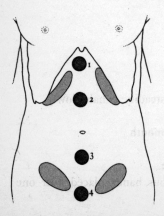

1 solar plexus
2 upper intestinal plexus
3 lower intestinal plexus
4 plexus of the lower abdomen

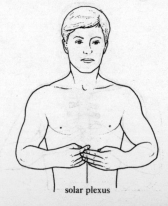

solar plexus

Hook your fingers under your right ribs.

- apply gentle pressure, slowly and deeply, to calm the area; exhale
- maintain the pressure for a few moments and breathe naturally
- gradually relax the pressure; inhale slowly and deeply
- after a series of 10 applications, reverse the procedure for the other side.

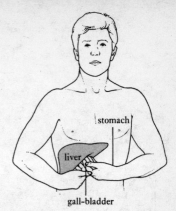

2   Overall relief of tension and stress

Sit down and let your arms encircle your bent knees.

- exert pressure on your abdomen and chest by bringing your knees up with the help of your arms; exhale
- relax; inhale.

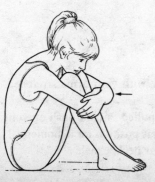

This exercise exerts pressure on the throat, abdomen and chest. It also improves the circulation to the upper half of your back and its nervous pathways which control your heart, respiration and digestion.

Lie down and raise your pelvis with the help of your elbows on the floor and your hands on your back. Let your legs remain relaxed and make sure your neck is not under excessive pressure.

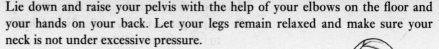

- tilt your body further by pushing gently on the lumbar area; exhale
- relax; inhale
- repeat the exercise 10 times
- bring your body back to the floor and stretch out; inhale deeply.

// *Strengthening exercises*

1 To improve the mobility of the throat

Place the palms of your hands flat on your knees, with your arms stretched, and open your mouth.
- inhale as you raise your chest with your chin pulled in, and push on your hands to accentuate the inhalation; maintain this position for a moment
- relax the contracted muscles at the front of your neck; exhale
- repeat the exercise 10 times.

2 To improve the performance of the respiratory muscles

This exercise stimulates the pectoral muscles in particular.

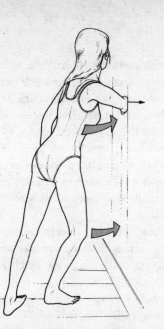

Stand sideways on to a wall, with the palm of your right hand on the wall at chest height, fingers pointing forwards. Put your legs slightly apart and put your right foot forward.

● bring the weight of your body towards the wall by bending your right leg – this will stretch your pectoral muscles; inhale
● relax; exhale
● after a series of 10 movements, reverse the procedure for the other side
● repeat the exercise with your left hand placed first at face height, then level with the top of your head. In this way you stretch each group of muscles in your chest.

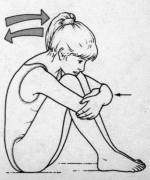

3 To help the abdomen to relax and to improve the circulation in the back

Sit down and let your arms encircle your bent knees.
● let yourself roll backwards; exhale
● come forwards to a sitting position again; inhale
● repeat the exercise 10 times.

Stress and irritability

'I'm under too much stress' is a common complaint today. It may be stress from all the travelling to and fro we do every day, stress from our jobs, from taxes, setbacks, competition, our family, joy, sadness . . . or just boredom. It's with us when we go to bed and it's with us when we get up. But who is this companion who sticks to us like glue and makes our life so unbearable?

Stress is above all a feeling of being always in a hurry and 'under pressure'. This is coupled with the inner tension we feel when we are faced with external situations which involve us whether we like it or not. We have to struggle not to let ourselves be overcome by it all, pushed aside and isolated in a world which continually seems to jostle and knock us about.

Many of us live in a state of permanent tension, with our nerves on edge, unable to relax and savour life's good moments. Stress makes us smoke and drink much more than we should, eat unhealthily, or make decisions which we regret later. Stress impedes our breathing, raises our blood-pressure and makes our heart race. We become prone to a whole variety of minor illnesses that come and go until finally we develop something really serious.

How can we put one face to this many-faceted, insidious, intangible illness we call stress? The key to stress, just like that of well-being, lies within our autonomic nervous system, which is so essential to life.

The collection of exercises in this book will help relieve all these harmful manifestations and give us back the time and space to live.

I   Exercises for relief

1   To relieve tension in the back and shoulders

Lean forward with your hands against a wall, a piece of furniture or a door-frame
at chest height, and your legs stretched slightly apart so that your back is flat.
● let your chest drop lightly; inhale
● let your back spring up again; exhale
● repeat the exercise 10 times.

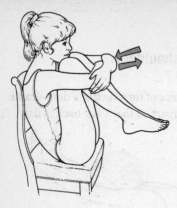

Sit on a chair or on the ground; let your arms encircle your bent knees, then put your chin between your knees.

● bring your knees up to your chest; exhale
● move your knees away from your chest; inhale
● repeat the exercise 10 times.

Kneel down with your back flat, your arms stretched out in front of you, and your forehead on the floor.

● unfold and stretch your body, with your chin raised towards the ceiling and your arms stretched and bearing your weight, and without arching your back too much; inhale
● bring your buttocks backwards and flatten your back, without moving your hands; exhale
● repeat the exercise 10 times.

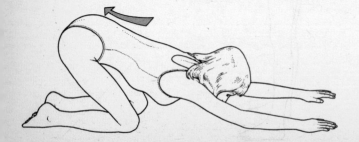

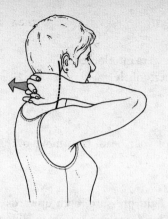

2   To relieve tension in the neck and shoulders

This tension is constant and makes the whole of our body tight. Improve the circulation to the muscles of the neck and shoulders by applying pressure to these muscles.

Put your hands around the back of your neck with your arms relaxed.
- squeeze the muscles at the back of your neck, steadily increasing the pressure, by bringing the palms of your hands together; exhale
- maintain the pressure, breathing shallowly
- relax the pressure; inhale
- repeat the procedure 10 times
- operate along the whole of your neck.

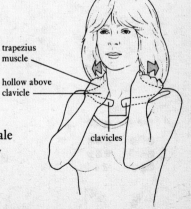

trapezius muscle

hollow above clavicle

clavicles

Lay the palm of each hand on the trapezius muscle at the top of your shoulders.
- apply pressure to the hollows above your shoulder-blades against the trapezius; exhale
- maintain the pressure, breathing shallowly
- relax the pressure; inhale
- repeat the procedure 10 times.

For other exercises see *Tension in the neck and shoulders*, pp. 79–85.

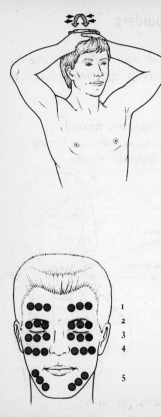

3   To relieve tension in the face and head

Place your hands on top of your head with your fingers interlocked.
- lift your scalp by bringing your palms together; inhale
- maintain the pressure and breathe naturally
- relax the pressure; exhale
- repeat the procedure 10 times
- work in the same manner along the centre of your head, then move over the whole of your scalp.

With the first three fingers of both hands apply light pressure, both upwards and downwards, at successive points across your head, making your skin slide over the bone.
- breathe naturally
- repeat 10 times in each of the following areas:
  1 along your forehead
  2 just under your brows
  3 along the lower edge of your eye-sockets
  4 under your cheek-bones
  5 on your chin
  6 in the hollows of your temples (a very sensitive area)
  7 above your jaw-bone, in front of your ear (very sensitive)
  8 under the occipital bone at the back of your neck.

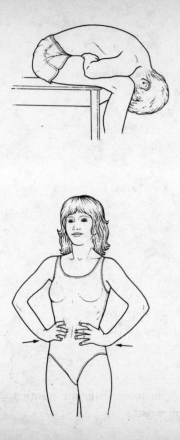

4   To relieve tension at the solar plexus

This tension is almost permanent.

Sit down and bend forward with your head between your legs, your arms bent and resting on your thighs, and your fingers placed over each other at the pit of your stomach, under the point of your sternum.

- apply careful pressure to the area around your solar plexus, stopping before it becomes painful; exhale, deflating your abdomen
- maintain the pressure for a few moments, breathing shallowly
- inhale, swelling out your abdomen and relaxing the pressure steadily
- repeat the exercise 10 times.

5   To improve the oxygen supply

Abdominal muscles

Put your hands on your hips, above your pelvis.
- squeeze while exhaling
- maintain the pressure and breathe naturally
- maintain some pressure as you inhale
- hold your breath at the end of the inhalation
- repeat the exercise 10 times.

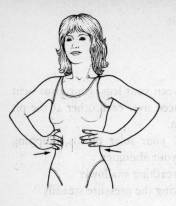

Diaphragm muscle

Put your hands on your lower ribs.
- apply careful pressure, taking care not to injure your ribs; exhale
- maintain the pressure and breathe shallowly
- relax the pressure; inhale
- repeat the exercise 10 times.

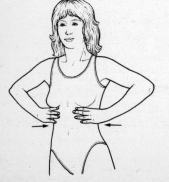

Intercostal muscles

Place both hands over your ribs, some distance from your armpits.
- apply pressure carefully as you exhale
- maintain the pressure and breathe naturally
- maintain some pressure while inhaling
- repeat the exercise 10 times.

This exercise can be practised with your hands in more than one position, according to the suppleness of your shoulders and wrists.

//   *Strengthening exercises*

1   Redistributing the circulation

In times of stress we tend to tense the same groups of muscles. A simple change from an upright to a lying position results in a change in blood-pressure and distribution of the blood, without the constraint of gravity. The supply of blood to the internal organs will also be modified. Practising exercises in unaccustomed but comfortable positions uses different nerves, helps reduce physical tenseness and produces a feeling of bodily harmony and well-being.

Exercise involving the sides of the body

Lie on your side with your right arm bent, your right hand under your head and your left arm relaxed. Then put your left hand on the floor in front of you with your legs relaxed and bent.

- raise your head and both legs at the same time, with the help of a push from your left hand and right elbow; exhale
- return to the ground; inhale
- repeat the exercise 10 times.

A leg exercise which stretches the body downwards

Lie on your back with your hands under your neck, your feet apart on the ground, your legs bent and your knees together.
● push simultaneously on the ground with your feet and forwards with your knees so that you stretch your lower back; inhale
● relax and come down to the ground; exhale
● repeat the exercise 10 times.
Be careful not to arch the bottom of your back too much, and to keep your head and feet in the same spot.

Exercise involving the arms, legs and back

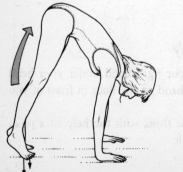

Go down on all fours, with your legs and arms stretched and your back parallel with the ground; bring your hands towards your feet until you feel a slight tension in your leg muscles.
● push your buttocks backwards to accentuate the tension in your legs; exhale, and lower your heels to the ground
● let your buttocks spring forwards again so that you feel some tension in your arms; inhale, and lift your heels off the ground.

Lean forward with your hands against the wall at chest height, and place your legs so that your back is flat.

- raise your chin towards the ceiling and arch your body slightly; inhale, and feel the tension in your outstretched arms
- bring your buttocks forwards again and flatten your back, without moving your hands; exhale
- repeat the exercise 10 times.

2 To improve respiration

Lie down on your back, bend your legs, and put your knees together, your feet apart and your arms on the ground beside your body.

- move your arms upwards along the ground, trying not to lose contact with the ground; inhale slowly
- when your arms are above your head, interlock your fingers and turn the palms of your hands over to stretch more; continue to inhale as deeply as possible, and feel the bottom of your back hollowing and your chin coming down towards your neck
- bring your clasped hands and your arms, relaxed and bent, down to your chest; exhale slowly, and feel the bottom of your back descending to the floor and your chin and head rocking backwards.

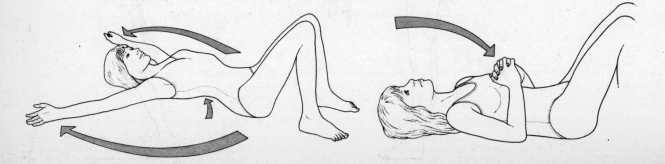

3   To improve the blood supply to the autonomic nervous centres and pathways in the back

The nervous pathways responsible for the heart and for respiration start at the top of the back.

Lie with your buttocks against a wall, with your feet placed on the wall and your hands on your knees.

- push simultaneously on the wall with your feet and on your knees with your hands so that you lift your body gradually off the ground, starting with your lower back, inhale slowly
- pause with the weight on the top part of your back for a few moments and breathe shallowly
- relax the pressure gradually so that you bring your buttocks down to the ground; exhale as they come down.

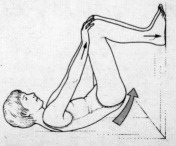

Feeling low and nervous depression

After a series of traumatic events, one more upset can make us feel really low. Sometimes a single blow is enough: the loss of a loved one, a painful separation, an emotional upheaval, a setback in our professional life, retirement coupled with fear of growing old, or financial problems. A weariness with life may overwhelm us; we feel completely helpless, misunderstood, rejected, and abandoned. Everything seems to be going wrong. Things go from bad to worse in all spheres of our life, and we are finally left exhausted, irritable, and indifferent to everything.

For many men, their anxieties focus on their professional and financial problems – they find it difficult to feel they are 'real men' if they are unable to earn a decent living. Economic crises, international competition, uncertainty about the future, fear of redundancy or unemployment predisposes many of them to depression. For the average woman, it is emotional conflicts that seem to affect her most deeply; but the constraints under which many women live in both their professional and their family lives explain why even a 'super-woman' can sometimes feel low.

Other groups who are particularly prone to depression are immigrants and people of rural origin who feel isolated in big towns, those with a serious physical illness or other disability, and those in a continual state of anxiety.

People who are depressed suffer from low morale and a feeling of unrelievable sadness. They are also prone to other problems, such as insomnia, lack of appetite, loss of weight, constipation, sexual problems and loss of libido, physical and mental lassitude with a diminution of memory and concentration and an incapacity for taking the initiative. Alcoholism, leaving home and various kinds of incoherent behaviour are common. In extreme cases there is a risk of suicide, in which case medical opinion should be sought.

It is possible to help ourselves, however, to avert these experiences. In addition to finding comfort and support from friends, family or professionals, we can try to improve the nervous condition of our bodies with some exercises.

/ *Exercises for relief*

1 To improve the respiration

When we are extremely depressed we feel a bit like a tyre that's been deflated. We know we need to take in more air, for we are suffering from a critical lack of it, yet breathing sometimes demands an effort which makes us feel even more exhausted. Our nervous system, which is particularly affected during a bout of depression, is maintained essentially by the oxygen in the air. If we cannot reawaken the respiratory process which aerates our body, the depression will persist and jeopardize our body's return to vital equilibrium.

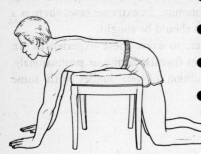

Go down on all fours and rest your chest on a cushion placed on a chair, with your arms hanging loose and your legs relaxed.

● make use of the involuntary inhalation reflex which forces the lungs to remain for a few moments without breath

● empty your lungs as much as possible and stay as long as you can without breathing

● as soon as you feel the need for air, half open your mouth to inhale involuntarily, without moving

● repeat the procedure 10 times.

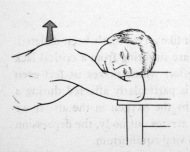

Sit down, bend your elbows and rest them on a desk, with your hands lying flat on top of one another and your head turned to one side. Rest your cheek on your hands. Stretch your back and shoulders and push your buttocks well to the back of your chair.

● exhale slowly and completely, then stop breathing, close your mouth tightly and feel your back getting flatter

● as soon as you feel the need for air, half open your mouth to inhale involuntarily, without moving, then feel your back grow round as the air enters your lungs

● repeat the procedure 10 times.

2 To improve the circulation

Use the same starting position as in the first exercise in this section (i.e. on all fours across a chair), and give yourself a gentle 'thoracic massage' by squeezing your chest with a regular rhythm.
- push down on your hands; inhale
- let your body fall on to the cushion; exhale
- repeat the exercise until you feel your body warming up.

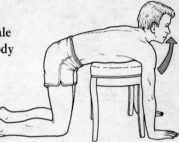

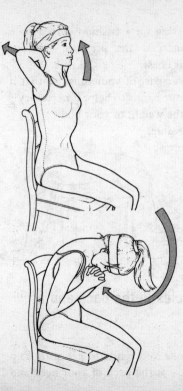

Sit on a chair and bring your hands, clasped together, to the back of your neck, with your arms relaxed and your legs together.
- take your head and elbows backwards; inhale slowly
- bring your hands, still clasped, over your head and squeeze your rib cage with your elbows; exhale completely
- as soon as you feel the need for air, bring your clasped hands to the back of your neck again; inhale calmly
- repeat the exercise 10 times.

3 To improve the functioning of the digestive tract

Go down on all fours, with your abdomen resting on a cushion placed on a
chair and your legs half stretched out to increase the pressure on your
abdomen. Stretch your arms out to hold up your chest.

- inhale, and take the air down into the lower part of your lungs so that it
  swells out your abdomen; push down on your hands to help, if necessary
- exhale, and let your chest be squeezed by the weight of your body
- remain without breathing for as long as possible,
  before inhaling again and repeating the exercise
- repeat the exercise 10 times.

4 To relax and loosen up all the muscles in the back and at the back of the neck

When you are depressed, your body has no tone and tends to get stiff. You
ache all over, especially at the base of your back, at the back of your neck and

in your shoulders. This is only logical, since these areas control our upright posture.

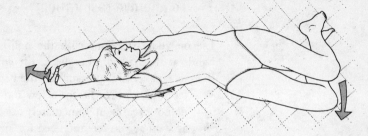

Lie flat on the floor on your back, with your legs bent and your hands together above your head.

- let your knees descend together to the right and stretch your arms to the left; inhale
- bring back your knees, still bent, to the centre; exhale
- let your knees descend together to the left and stretch your arms to the right; inhale
- bring your knees back again to the centre; exhale
- repeat the exercise 10 times.

This exercise stretches the dorsal muscles in a gentle but progressive way. It pushes the body quite naturally towards the feet. Allow your neck and head to follow the movements of your body.

// *Strengthening exercises*

1 To improve respiration

Lie on your back and with the help of your elbows on the floor and your hands at the base of your back, lift your pelvis; relax your legs, making sure there is no excessive pressure on the back of your neck.

● let yourself breathe for a few moments in this position; then exhale and do not breathe in immediately
● as soon as you feel the need for air, bring your pelvis down to the ground as you inhale
● continue to inhale as you stretch the whole of your body
● repeat the exercise 10 times.

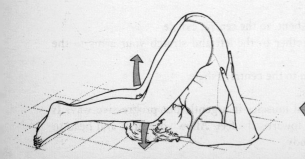

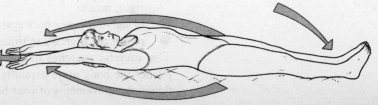

2   To improve the blood supply to the back

This exercise benefits the back muscles as well as the nervous pathways issuing from the spinal cord.

Lie on your back and put your buttocks against a wall, with your feet resting on the wall and your hands on your knees.
- push simultaneously on the wall with your feet and on your knees with your hands, so that you raise your body gradually off the ground; inhale
- pause for a few moments on any tender area, and breathe naturally
- bring your buttocks down to the ground; exhale
- repeat the exercise 10 times.

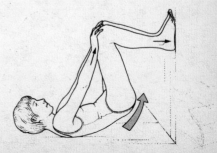

3 To improve the circulation

Exercising the legs helps the blood flow from the heart to the extremities and improves their circulation.

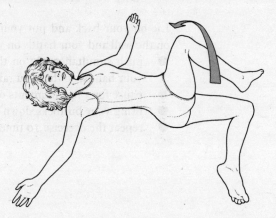

Lie on your back, with your arms stretched out horizontally and your left leg bent and lying so that its outer side faces the ground.
- throw your right leg over your left leg; exhale
- let your right leg spring back to a neutral position; inhale
- repeat the exercise until you feel your body warming up
- after a series of 10 movements, reverse the procedure for the other side.

URINARY PROBLEMS

Cystitis

Sufferers from cystitis usually feel a sharp burning sensation as they pass urine, or, despite a strong urge to urinate frequently, produce only a few drops.

Women often get cystitis after childbirth or a vaginal infection. Colitis, constipation, infections and diseases of the kidneys and urinary tract can also cause it, as can stress from personal relationships.

/ *Exercises for relief*

1 To soothe irritation in the lower abdomen

Lie down on your back with your legs bent, your knees together and your feet apart; place your hands above your pubis.

- apply pressure to your lower abdomen and increase it slowly; exhale
- maintain the pressure and breathe shallowly
- relax the pressure gradually; inhale
- repeat the treatment 10 times
- repeat the treatment to the lower intestinal plexus and the adjacent areas.

VARIATION: Do the same exercise in the other positions (see pp. 50–53).

2 To improve respiration

Kneel down with your arms half bent above your head and your forehead on the ground. Put your buttocks on your heels with the upper surface of your feet on the ground or your feet bent over your toes.

- swell out your abdomen slowly and inhale slowly
- deflate your abdomen gradually and exhale slowly
- repeat the exercise 10 times.

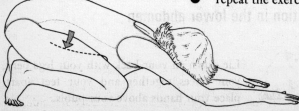

// *Strengthening exercises*

1   To improve the blood supply to the nervous pathways

Lie down on your back sufficiently far away from a wall to rest your feet against it, with your legs very slightly bent and your hands on top of each other on your abdomen.
● push against the wall with your right foot and exhale
● push on the wall with your left foot; inhale, and feel the pressure on your sacrum at the base of your spine
● repeat the exercise 10 times.

Use the same position as in the last exercise.
● rock your knees and pelvis to the right without moving the position of your feet on the wall; inhale
● return to the starting position; exhale, and feel the pressure on your sacrum
● after a series of 10 movements, reverse the procedure for the other side.

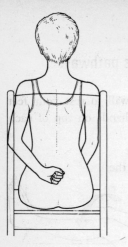

Sit on a chair and place your left fist between your back and the chair-back at the level of your sacrum.
- lean back so that you squeeze your sacrum; inhale
- maintain the pressure and breathe shallowly
- come forward again to release the pressure; exhale
- repeat the exercise 10 times.

2 To improve respiration

Go down on all fours.
- make your back rounded and bring your head down into your chest; exhale

- raise your head and lift your chin up as high as possible, while your back arches (though not too much); inhale, and feel the stretching in the front of your chest and abdomen
- repeat the exercise 10 times.

Stress incontinence

Sometimes when you cough, sneeze, or burst out laughing, you involuntarily pass some urine without having felt the need to do so. Sometimes you experience this incontinence as you stand up.

Incontinence is usually caused by damage to the vesical sphincter, which can be torn in childbirth, or by a prolapse of the bladder, vagina or rectum. But it may also affect older people who cannot control their sphincters properly. This causes them a good deal of embarrassment in their everyday lives.

The retraining of the pelvic muscles is always beneficial, either to avoid the necessity of surgery, which is often the only solution to incontinence, or before and after a corrective operation, and following childbirth.

Exercises for relief and to strengthen the system

1   The muscles of the pelvic floor (muscles closing the bottom of the pelvis)

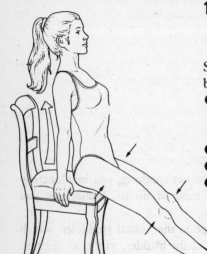

Sit on the edge of a chair, with your arms stretched downwards, resting on the back of a chair-seat, and your legs stretched out in front of you.

- squeeze together your feet, knees, thighs and buttocks; inhale slowly and stretch your body slightly backwards, increasing the inhaling action; try to control your pelvic muscles
- relax; exhale
- repeat the exercise 10 times
- reverse the position of your legs and repeat the exercise.

This exercise is similar to the previous one, allowing you passively to prevent any descent of your organs within your body. Lie on your back with your legs stretched out against a wall at some height from the ground. Place one foot above the other with your hands on your thighs.

- squeeze together your feet, knees, thighs and buttocks – this stretches your body; inhale slowly, and practise controlling the pelvic muscles which contract at the same time
- relax; exhale
- repeat the exercise 10 times
- reverse the position of your legs and repeat the exercise.

2   Breathing

The aim is to alleviate pressure within the abdomen. Any exercise which improves chest expansion by controlling the muscles of the buttocks and the pelvis will help cure incontinence.

Lie on your front, leaning on your elbows with your legs apart.
- draw back your head and press down on your elbows; inhale slowly and deeply, while squeezing your buttocks and your pelvic muscles
- lower your head again; exhale
- repeat the exercise 10 times.

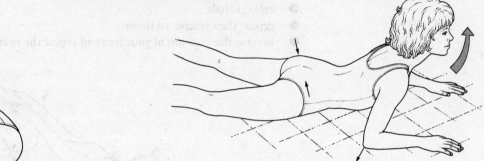

Lie on your right side with your right arm bent under your head, your left arm stretched out in front, and your legs bent on top of each other.
- extend your left leg and take it in an arc backwards, sliding your left foot along the ground; inhale slowly and deeply and feel the muscles in your buttocks and hips contracting
- keeping your left leg stretched, bring it back in an arc to the front; exhale
- after a series of 10 movements, reverse the procedure for the other side.

Kneel in front of a chair with your hands on the chair-seat, your knees apart, and the weight of your body on your heels.

- raise your pelvis and lift your chin towards the ceiling, so that your back arches slightly; inhale slowly and deeply and feel the muscles in your buttocks and pelvis contracting
- return to the starting position and exhale
- repeat the exercise 10 times.

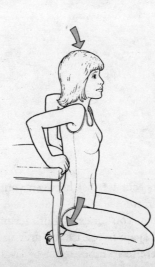 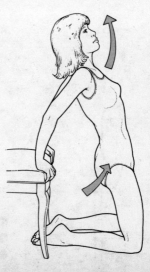

3 The autonomic nervous system

Lie on your back and take hold of your knees with your hands or your arms.
- roll backwards; exhale
- roll forwards; inhale
- repeat the exercise 10 times.

Make sure you roll on your sacrum.

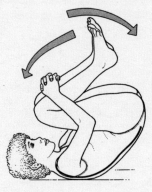

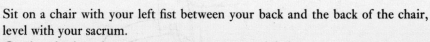

Sit on a chair with your left fist between your back and the back of the chair, level with your sacrum.
- lean back so that you squeeze your sacrum; inhale
- come forward again to release the pressure; exhale
- repeat the exercise 10 times.

Tendency to kidney-stones

Those who have experienced passing a kidney-stone never forget the violent pain it brings to the lumbar region, spreading out towards the thighs and genital area. No position seems to bring relief, and in the end the pain is so excruciating that we just can't keep still for a moment. This renal colic is often accompanied by vomiting, a distended abdomen, pain when passing urine and general distress. An attack can last several hours, until the stone is expelled into the bladder. Sometimes the pain may resemble a bout of sciatica or lumbago; on other occasions it can seem like appendicitis, a perforated ulcer or even a coronary thrombosis.

Attacks often occur after a journey, a period of intense fatigue, eating too much or drinking alcohol. They are caused when what is often a very small kidney-stone blocks the urinary passages. It is the resulting spasm and oedema (local swelling), however, which brings on the intolerable pain, and only urgent medical treatment prevents damage to the kidneys.

If sufferers can manage to drink enough water to prevent the formation of further kidney-stones, they can also improve their urinary output with some special exercises. We should remember that most of us do not drink enough fluid every day to eliminate our body wastes effectively. This leaves us sooner or later exposed to kidney problems, with overwork and ageing as complementary causes. On average we should take in $1\frac{1}{2}$–2 litres of liquid a day, preferably in the form of mineral water. This corresponds to 6–8 large glassfuls, which sounds a lot but is easy enough to drink if we spread it over intervals of $1\frac{1}{2}$–2 hours throughout the day. And don't forget that as well as easing the passage of urine, drinking also renews the water content of our body cells. After air, it is water that our body needs most.

/ *Exercises for relief*

We should take the same measures as we do for a pain in the lumbar region or on the right side of the abdomen, except in the case of an acute bout of pain.

1   To calm abdominal spasm

Lie down on your back, with the upper part of your body raised to help the flow of urine and maybe of a kidney-stone. With the fingers of both hands touching on the side where the pain is, bend your legs to relax the abdominal wall and put your knees together and your feet apart.

● exhale, while sinking the fingers of both hands steadily deeper into the top right-hand part of your abdomen
● maintain the pressure for a few moments; inhale, steadily relaxing the pressure

- repeat the treatment 10 times over the right-hand part of the abdomen
- finish by applying the same kind of pressure above your pubis to help empty your bladder.

Lie on your back so that your thighs are at a right angle to your abdomen and calves, with your feet on the wall, your right hand flat under your lumbar region, and your left arm lying along your body.

- gently rock your knees to the right, letting your feet remain in the same place; exhale, and feel the pressure of your hand against your lower back
- stay in this position for a few moments, maintaining the pressure and breathing shallowly
- bring your knees back to their starting position; inhale, and feel the pressure taken off your lower back
- repeat the treatment over your lumbar region and sacrum.

This exercise not only relaxes the muscles at the base of your back, but also improves the blood supply to the nervous pathways controlling the passage of urine.

VARIATION: Sit on a chair, placing a fist between your back and the chair-back.
● lean back so that you apply some pressure; inhale
● maintain the pressure, breathing shallowly
● come forward again to release the pressure; exhale
● repeat the exercise 10 times.

3   Improving respiration

Improving our breathing gives the diaphragm muscle more work, and this in turn helps to relax the region of the abdomen that is in spasm. It also improves the circulation by encouraging the return of venous blood to the heart. The first exercise has several advantages. It helps you to massage your back by means of the wall, and it encourages the relaxation of the sphincters in the lower section of your body and the elimination of urine.

Crouch down with your back against a wall and your
hands on your knees.
- lean forward, rolling your body into a ball; exhale
- bring your trunk up again by pressing on your
  knees with your hands; inhale deeply
- repeat the exercise 10 times.

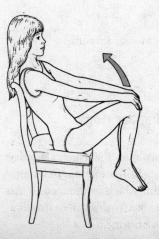

Sit against the back of a chair, with your hands clasping your knees.
- bring your knees up to your chest; exhale
- lower them again and stretch your arms; inhale
- repeat the exercise 10 times.

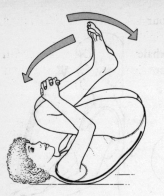

// *Strengthening exercises*

1 To improve the blood supply to the lumbar and sacral regions

This is important for the nervous pathways which control the kidneys and the elimination of urine.

Sit on the floor, with your arms encircling your bent knees.
- let yourself roll backwards; exhale
- let yourself come back forwards; inhale

Take care to roll particularly on your lumbar area and your sacrum.

2 To improve the working of the dorso-lumbar ridge

The region where the concave dorsal curve turns into the convex lumbar curve is one of the most important in the body. Stiffening up frequently occurs here, reducing the mobility of the diaphragm, which is attached to this point, and impairing the blood supply to the nervous pathways controlling, among other things, kidney function.

Kneel down with your buttocks raised, your arms stretched along the ground on either side of your head, and your face resting on the ground.

● push your buttocks back without allowing your arms to lose contact with the ground; exhale, feeling the whole of your back stretching and your lumbar region hollowing out naturally

● bring your buttocks forward and let your head roll to one side; inhale, and feel your back and particularly your lumbar area becoming rounded

● repeat the exercise 10 times.

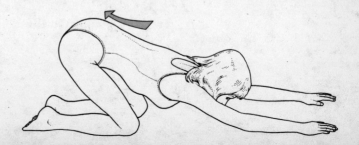

Take hold of the uprights of a door-frame at chest height, with your feet at a distance of about 3 feet from the wall, and push your buttocks backwards while holding on with your hands.

- slightly bend your right knee; exhale, and feel your left side stretching
- stretch your right knee; inhale
- after a series of 10 movements, reverse the procedure for the other side.

Be careful when you stand up straight: first of all stoop down, then bring yourself up by pushing on your knees with your hands.

3   To strengthen the muscles involved in twisting the trunk

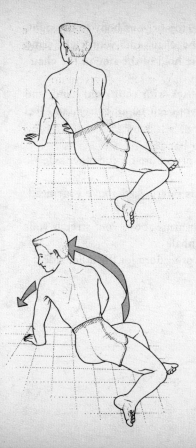

These muscles stop those in the lower back and the dorso–lumbar ridge area from seizing up. They consist mainly of the abdominal muscles. Their elasticity prevents any digestive or circulatory stoppage, and has an indirect but important influence on the regulation of nerves and the circulation to all the abdominal organs.

Sit on the ground and bend your right leg with its inside surface to the floor; bend your left leg with its outside surface to the floor, and put your left foot against your right knee. Place your hands on the ground to the left behind you, with your arms stretched.

● bend your trunk back a little further and to the left by lowering your left elbow and shoulder; exhale

● return to the starting position; inhale

● after a series of 10 movements, reverse the procedure for the other side.

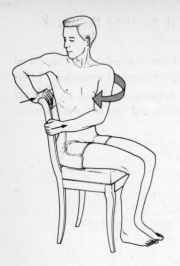

Sit on a chair with your legs together. Turn the top of your body to the right, with your right shoulder over the back of the chair and your right hand resting on the chair-back; let your left hand take hold of the side of the chair-back.

● simultaneously (a) push against the chair-back with your right hand, and (b) pull the chair-back towards you with your left hand; exhale, and feel the twist in all your trunk muscles

● return to the starting position; inhale

● after a series of 10 movements, reverse the procedure for the other side.

Lie on your back, with the fingers of both hands interlocked above your head. Bend your legs and tilt over to your right side.

● turn your head to the left and stretch your arms above you; stretch your thighs by pushing down with your knees; inhale

● after a series of 10 movements, reverse the procedure for the other side.

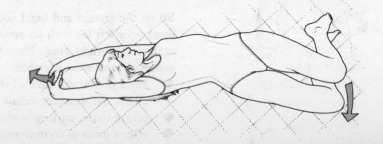

4   To improve respiration

Sit down with your legs apart, your left elbow on your left knee, and your right arm above your head.
- stretch your right arm; inhale
- relax; exhale
- after a series of 10 movements, reverse
  the procedure for the other side.

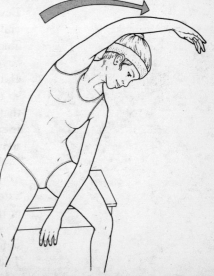

GYNAECOLOGICAL PROBLEMS

Painful periods

Few women are lucky enough to have pain-free menstruation during their childbearing years. Some experience simply a heavy feeling or an uncomfortable contraction in their lower abdomen at this time of the month, but others have to endure severe pain in the genital area, which spreads to the lower back and puts a stop to any activity for the time being. The unluckiest ones may be so unwell, with unpleasant symptoms such as nausea, vomiting or headache, that they have to stay in bed. They are unable to cope with domestic, professional and social commitments, they miss job opportunities and parties, and some even fail exams!

Why do women suffer this way? In most cases the unpleasant symptoms can be explained by the body: hormonal imbalance, hyperactivity of the autonomic nervous system controlling the genital sphere, circulatory problems, or the action of a hormone known as prostoglandin on uterine contractions. In a very small proportion of cases, the regularity of the problem arises from some organic damage, such as a genital infection or a gynaecological disease. There can also be psychological causes.

/ *Exercises for relief*

1   To calm spasmodic contractions

Direct treatment to the plexus of the lower abdomen, then to the autonomic nervous pathways emerging from the sacrum, is usually effective. Proceed carefully and gently.

Lie on the floor with your legs bent, your knees together and your feet apart; place the fingers of both hands just above your pubis, level with your bladder, which should previously have been emptied.

- apply pressure, increasing it gradually; exhale
- maintain the pressure for a few moments and breathe shallowly
- steadily relax the pressure; inhale
- repeat the procedure 10 times.

Lie on the floor some distance from a wall, with your legs slightly bent, your feet on the wall and your arms relaxed and lying on the floor.
● push your feet against the wall; inhale
● feel the pressure on your sacrum, and your pelvis rocking slightly
● stop pushing but do not move your feet; exhale
● repeat the exercise, pushing first on one foot and then on the other (walking on the spot on the wall); inhale and exhale alternately.

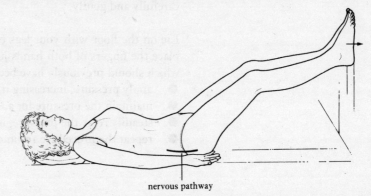

nervous pathway

VARIATION: Sit down with your fist between your back and the back of a chair so that you apply pressure to the same areas.

2   To soothe pains in the lumbar region

Lie down some distance from a wall so that your legs are slightly bent and your feet rest on the wall. Place your right hand under your right lumbar area and your left hand on the ground.

- rock your legs slightly to the left; inhale
- bring your knees to the right – this will squeeze your lumbar area against your right hand; exhale
- repeat the exercise 10 times
- reverse the procedure for the other side.

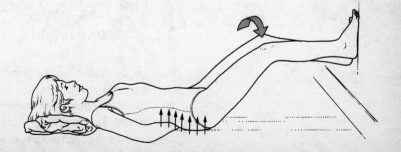

Kneel down with your arms out in front, your forehead on the ground; and your feet flat on the ground or raised on the toes.
- bring your thighs down to your heels without moving your forearms or hands; exhale
- relax and raise your thighs slightly; inhale, and let your forehead move over the floor
- repeat the exercise 10 times.

For other exercises, see *Pains in the lumbar area*, pp. 86–101.

3   To improve respiration

Position yourself as in the previous exercise. Relax your abdominal muscles to enable venous blood to return to your heart easily.
- inhale, swelling your abdomen
- exhale, deflating your abdomen
- repeat the exercise 10 times.

Place your hands, with fingers interlocked, on the crown of your head.

● stretch your arms, turning the palms of your hands outwards and towards the ceiling; inhale, and feel the stretching right up to your fingers
● bring your hands down to your head; exhale
● repeat the exercise 10 times.

// *Strengthening exercises*

1 To exercise the pelvic muscles

Kneel down, with your hands placed in front of you and your arms stretched.

● sway over to the right so that you are sitting on your right buttock; exhale
● return to the position you started in; inhale
● sway over to the left so that you are sitting on your left buttock; exhale
● repeat the exercise 10 times.

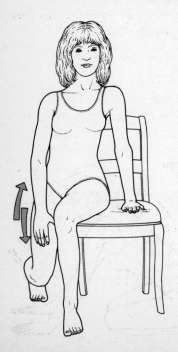

Sit on the side of a chair so that your left buttock rests on the chair and your right one is off it. Place your left hand on the chair to maintain your balance, with your right arm on your right thigh.

- shift your body weight on to your right buttock, which is off the chair; exhale
- bring your body weight on to your left buttock, making your right buttock rise; inhale
- after a series of 10 movements, reverse the procedure for the other side.

Go down on all fours, with your knees slightly apart, your hands on the floor the width of your shoulders apart, and your arms stretched.

● simultaneously raise your chin towards the ceiling and push your buttocks slightly back; inhale, trying not to arch your back too much

● simultaneously (a) draw in your chin so that you look down towards your abdomen and (b) raise your pelvis towards your face; exhale

● repeat the exercise 10 times.

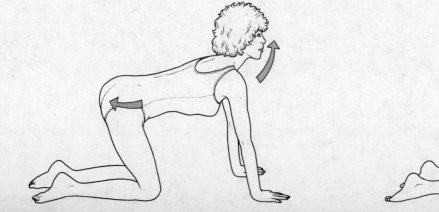
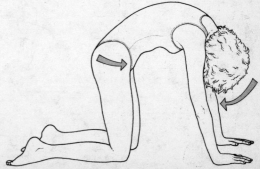

Kneel down in front of a chair, with your hands on the seat behind you, your knees apart and your buttocks on your heels.

● raise your pelvis and lift your chin up towards the ceiling, without arching your back too much; inhale
● lift yourself up by pushing on your hands
● come back on to your heels; exhale
● repeat the exercise 10 times.

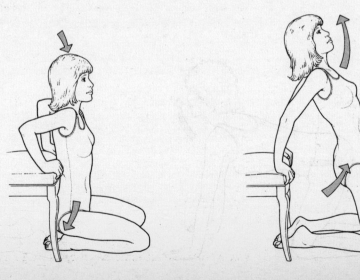

Sit on the floor with your legs together and stretched out in front of you, your hands placed on each side of your body, and your arms stretched.

- slightly bend your right knee and raise your right buttock, moving it a little bit further back; exhale, and 'walk' backwards with your buttocks
- put your right buttock on the floor; inhale, and move your right hand backwards as necessary
- bend your left knee and raise your left buttock, moving it backwards; exhale
- put your left buttock on the ground; inhale
- repeat the exercise 10 times.

VARIATION: Do the same exercise, walking forwards with the buttocks.

2 To exercise the abdominal and lumbar muscles

Lie on the ground and clasp your knees with your hands, leaving your legs relaxed and bent.

● bring your knees up to your chest with your hands; exhale
● push your knees back until your arms are stretched; inhale
● when the exercise becomes easy to do, practise it with your hands under your thighs, letting your feet fall to the ground
● repeat the exercise 10 times.

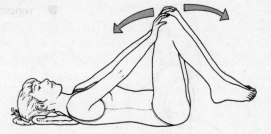

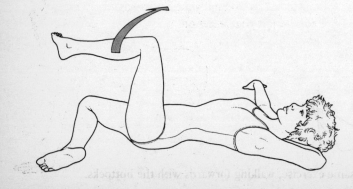

Lie down with your left arm bent and your hand under the back of your neck; stretch your right arm out to the side at right angles to your body, and bend your right knee with your foot on the ground.

- throw your left leg progressively further and further across your right leg without trying to stretch it; exhale
- let your left leg spring back to the central position; inhale
- after a series of 10 movements, reverse the procedure for the other side.

For other exercises, see *Pains in the lumbar area*, pp. 86–101.

3 To improve respiration

Get into a squatting position with your hands placed on the floor in front of you, the width of your shoulders apart, and your arms stretched.
Put your weight on your toes, and bring your head into your chest.
- push on your hands to help you to 'roll up' your body; exhale
- 'unroll' and, simultaneously, put your knees on the ground and raise your chin towards the ceiling; inhale
- repeat the exercise 10 times.

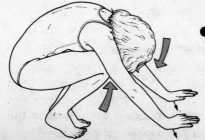

Premenstrual syndrome

This common condition affects one woman in three. A few days before a period is due her breasts swell and become very painful, her pelvis feels very heavy, her abdomen becomes distended and her digestion is upset. She may experience sleep disturbances and feel irritable. Other symptoms may include circulatory congestion and the failure of the body to eliminate fluids, which produces body and ankle puffiness and may add more than two kilos to the woman's body weight.

Your gynaecologist will probably explain that this bewildering assembly of problems can be caused by hormonal or circulatory factors, or be linked with nervous instability. He/she is quite likely to suggest that it's a matter of gritting your teeth and waiting for it to pass once your period begins.

/ Exercises for relief

1   To soothe tiredness and discomfort in the back

For the top half of the back

Lie on the ground with your buttocks against a wall, your feet resting on the wall and your hands on your knees.

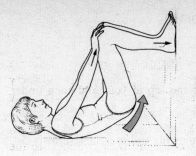

- push simultaneously on the wall with your feet and on your knees with your hands so that you raise your pelvis and then your back; inhale, and pause at each tender area
- slightly relax the pressure from your feet and hands; exhale
- push again with your hands and feet to find another tender area; inhale
- bring your buttocks down to the ground; exhale
- repeat the exercise 10 times.

For the bottom half of the back

Lie far enough away from a wall so that with your legs slightly bent you can put your feet on it; let your arms lie relaxed on the floor.

- push on the wall with your feet; inhale, feeling the pressure on your sacrum, then on your lumbar region, and feel your pelvis rocking slightly
- relax the pressure without moving your feet; exhale
- repeat the exercise 10 times.

VARIATION: Sit on a chair and put your fist or hand flat between your back and the chair-back so that you squeeze your back.

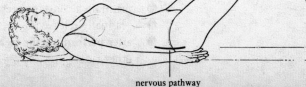

nervous pathway

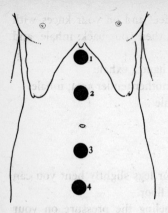

1 solar plexus
2 upper intestinal plexus
3 lower intestinal plexus
4 plexus of the lower abdomen

2 To reduce congestion in the abdomen

Pressure on the solar plexus

Put your fingers together and place them at the top of your abdomen under the point of your sternum.

● gradually increase the pressure; exhale
● maintain a constant pressure for a few moments and breathe shallowly
● gradually relax the pressure; inhale
● repeat the procedure on the other plexuses.

Pressure under the lower ribs on the right side

Hook your fingers under your right ribs.

● gradually increase the pressure so that you penetrate beneath your ribs, without going beyond a point where it becomes painful; exhale
● maintain a constant pressure for a few moments and breathe shallowly
● gradually release the pressure; inhale
● after performing the treatment 10 times, reverse the procedure for the other side.

3   To improve the circulation in the legs

Lie down, and put your right knee over your left knee with your legs bent and relaxed.

- draw your two bent knees towards your chest; exhale
- relax; inhale
- after a series of 10 movements, reverse the procedure for the other side.

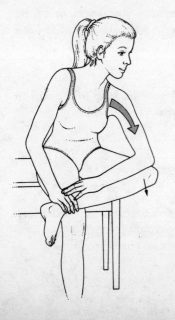

Put your left foot on your right knee, with your right hand on your left ankle, and your left forearm on your left leg.

- lean forward over your left knee; exhale, and feel the back of your left thigh stretching
- relax; inhale
- after a series of 10 movements, reverse the procedure for the other side.

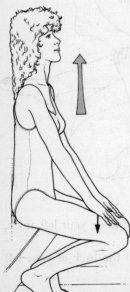

Squat with your back against a wall and your hands on your knees, looking straight ahead.

● helped by your hands pushing down on your knees, slide your back up the wall; inhale

● stand up straight, with your hands on the front of your thighs, looking straight ahead

● slowly slide your hands down your thighs as far as your knees, or a little lower, keeping your buttocks in contact with the wall; exhale, and feel the stretching in the back of your legs

● lean forwards with your hands on your knees

● raise your head and flatten your back; inhale

● slide your buttocks down the wall and bring your back up to the wall to finish in the position in which you started; exhale

● repeat the whole exercise 10 times.

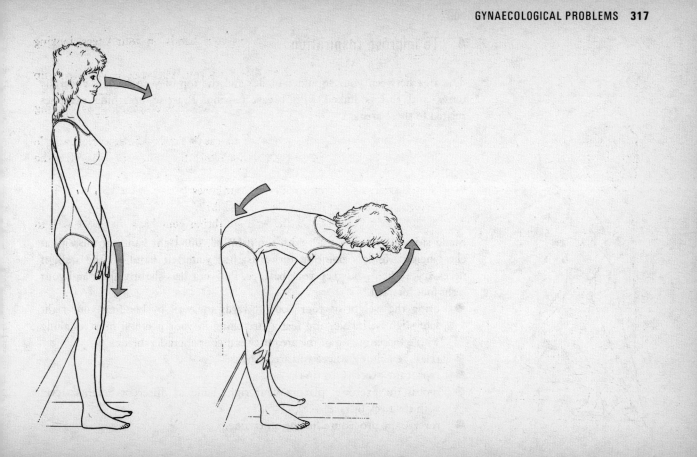

4   To improve respiration

The area between your shoulder-blades and the top of your back is generally tense, and this is linked with breast tension. Practise breathing exercises related to these areas.

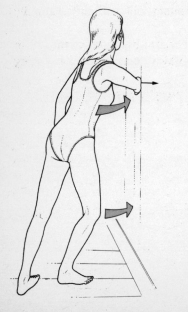

Stand sideways on to a wall, with the palm of your right hand on the wall at chest height, fingers pointing forwards; put your left hand on the wall, if necessary, to help you keep your balance. Put your legs slightly apart and your right foot forward.

● bring the weight of your body towards the wall by bending your right foot slightly; inhale, and feel a stretching in your pectoral muscles along with a loosening up of the area between your shoulder-blades

● relax, remaining where you are; exhale

● repeat the exercise 10 times

● repeat the exercise, placing your right hand at different heights (level with the neck or face)

● reverse the procedure for the other side.

Lie on your left side, with your right leg bent and relaxed over your relaxed left leg; let your relaxed arms lie along the ground to the left of your body, and lay your face on your left cheek.

● slide your right hand and your relaxed right arm to the right, describing an arc above your head; inhale, and feel a loosening at the top of your back and between your shoulder-blades; your head and the back of your neck will be carried along by the movement and will turn naturally towards the right

● slide your right hand and your relaxed right arm back over to the left in an arc above your head; exhale – in this way you return to the starting position

● after a series of 10 movements, reverse the procedure for the other side.

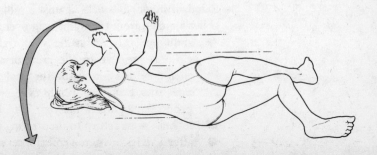

// *Strengthening exercises*

1 Exercises for loosening up the back

Stand with your buttocks against a wall, your legs slightly apart, and your feet about 8 inches from the wall. Lean over and let your arms hang loose.

● simultaneously (a) swing your right arm and right hand to the left as close as possible to the ground, and (b) bring your left elbow, which should be bent, towards the back; exhale, and feel a loosening in your hips, then bring the weight of your body on to your right leg, which will bend very slightly while your left leg stretches

● let both arms return to the starting position; inhale

● after a series of 10 movements, reverse the procedure for the other side.

2   Exercises for loosening up the legs

Stand with your hands some distance apart on the edge of a piece of furniture; bend your left knee, and stretch your right leg out well behind you.
● reverse the position of your legs by jumping and bringing your right foot forwards with your right knee bent, and your left foot to the rear with your left leg stretched; inhale while you jump
and exhale as your feet touch the ground again
● repeat the exercise 10 times.

Lie down and bend your right leg with your right foot on the ground; place your left foot on your right knee, letting your hands lie on your left thigh.

● push with both hands on your left thigh; inhale, and feel the inside of your thigh stretching
● relax; exhale
● after a series of 10 movements, reverse the procedure for the other side.

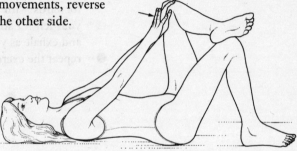

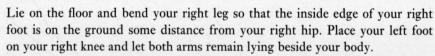

Lie on the floor and bend your right leg so that the inside edge of your right foot is on the ground some distance from your right hip. Place your left foot on your right knee and let both arms remain lying beside your body.

● press on your right knee with your left foot to push it down to the floor; inhale
● relax the pressure and let your knee spring back; exhale
● after a series of 10 movements, reverse the procedure for the other side.

3 To improve respiration

Lie across a bed and let your head hang over the edge. With your legs apart
and stretched out, let your arms relax and hang downwards.
● reach out with your hands towards the ground; inhale
● relax; exhale
● repeat the movement 10 times.

Pregnancy

Pregnancy is a major experience in a woman's life, and one which she should
be able to enjoy to the full. Some women experience a completely trouble-free
pregnancy, while others – and they are the majority – have many unpleasant symptoms in the first three months: for example, nausea, vomiting,
indigestion, and a frequent desire to pass urine, as well as irritability and dis-
turbed sleep. Later on, with the increase in their weight and the growing
size of their abdomen, women can suffer from back pain, particularly in the
lumbar region, tiredness in the legs, and breathlessness.

It would perhaps be a good idea if there were some kind of training course for pregnant women, to help their bodies adapt to the successive changes they must undergo during pregnancy – the redistribution of weight around the pelvis, the changes in blood circulation and breathing and in other bodily functions for example, which can all cause problems. Imagine what an outcry there would be from men if *they* were obliged steadily to increase the weight of their briefcases until they weighed some 30 lb!

1 To strengthen the belt of muscles in the lumbar and abdominal regions

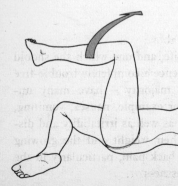

Lie on the ground with your right leg bent and resting on the ground, your left leg bent and carried over your right leg, and your left arm bent. Put your left hand under your neck, with your right arm lying on the ground at right angles to your body.

- bring your left leg gradually a little further to the right; exhale
- let your left leg spring back; inhale
- after a series of 10 movements, reverse the procedure for the other side.

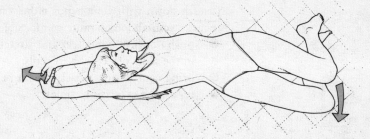

Lie on your back, with your fingers interlocked above your head, your legs bent and tilted over to the right, and your head turned to the left.
- simultaneously (a) stretch your arms to the left, and (b) stretch your thighs by pushing your knees to the right – if necessary, help the movement by pushing with your feet on the ground; inhale slowly and deeply
- relax and return to the starting position; exhale
- after a series of 10 movements, reverse the procedure for the other side.

For other exercises, see *Pains in the lumbar area*, pp. 86–101.

2 To strengthen the muscles in the legs

We should remember that if our thigh muscles are not working well we are more susceptible to pains in the lumbar region.

Crouch down with your hands either on the floor, or on a pile of thick books to make your abdomen more comfortable.
- push down on your feet and stretch your legs, while keeping your hands in the same place; inhale deeply
- bring your buttocks back to your heels; exhale
- repeat the exercise 10 times.

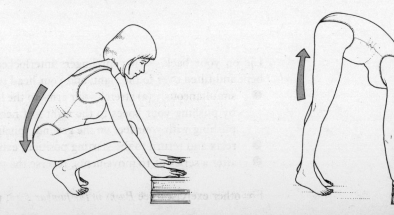

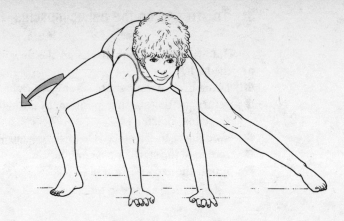

Go down on all fours, with your legs apart and stretched, your hands on the floor, and your arms stretched out in front of you.

- bend your right knee and bring the weight of your body on to your right leg; exhale, and feel your left leg stretching
- push down on your right foot so that you return to the starting position; inhale
- after a series of 10 movements, reverse the procedure for the other side.

VARIATION: Do the same exercise, putting your hands on a chair.

3   To strengthen the pelvic muscles

Kneel down and put your hands on the floor in front of you, with your arms stretched out.
- swing over to the right to sit on your right buttock; exhale
- return to the starting position by swinging your hips in the opposite direction; inhale
- swing over to the other side to sit on your left buttock; exhale
- return to the starting position; inhale
- repeat the exercise 10 times.

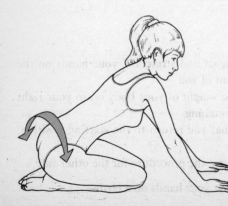

Go down on all fours, with your knees slightly apart on the ground, your hands placed on the ground the width of your shoulders apart, and your arms stretched.

● simultaneously (a) raise your chin towards the ceiling, and (b) push your buttocks slightly back; inhale, but be careful not to arch your back too much

● simultaneously (a) bring your chin into your chest so that you look down towards your abdomen, and (b) bring your hips towards your face, contracting your hip muscles; exhale

● repeat the exercise 10 times.

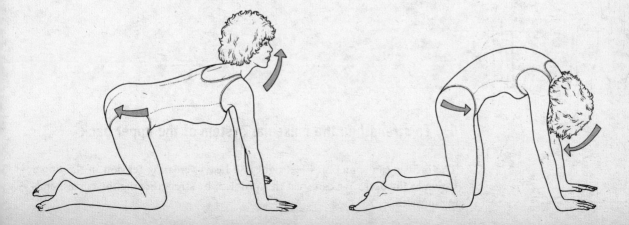

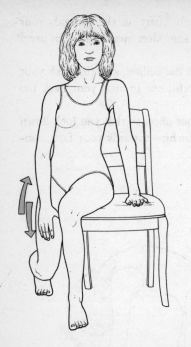

Sit on the edge of a chair so that your right buttock hangs over the edge and the left one rests on the seat. Place your left hand on the seat to maintain your balance, and put your right hand on your right thigh.

- let the weight of your body come on to your right buttock, which will sink towards the floor; exhale
- bring the weight of your body on to your left buttock to raise your right buttock again; inhale
- after a series of 10 movements, reverse the procedure for the other side.

4   To strengthen the muscular system of the upper back

The breasts can sometimes feel tight and heavy, creating tension in the upper region of the back. We can treat this problem by strengthening the corresponding muscles.

Rest your hands at shoulder level on a wall, a piece of furniture or a door-frame, with your legs apart and stretched. Place your feet some distance from the wall so that your back is flat.
- drop your chest while keeping your hands in the same place; inhale
- let your back spring up again; exhale
- repeat the exercise 10 times.

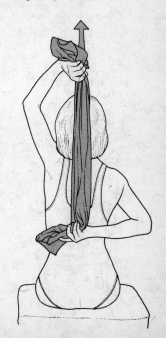

Sitting on a chair or standing up, hold a towel behind you as in the illustration.
- pull on the towel with your left hand; exhale, and let your right hand come up with the movement and accentuate the bending of your right arm
- pull on the towel with your right hand; inhale, and feel your left hand descend towards your left shoulder
- after a series of 10 movements, reverse the procedure for the other side.

5 To exercise the deep muscles of the pelvis

Sit on the edge of a chair and stretch your arms down, with your hands gripping the side of the seat for support. Stretch your legs out in front of you, one over the other.

● simultaneously squeeze your feet, your knees, your thighs and your buttocks; inhale slowly, and feel the contraction of your sphincter muscles and the deep muscular system of your pelvis – allow your body to stretch slightly backwards during the movement

● relax; exhale

● after a series of 10 movements, reverse the procedure for the other side.

Kneel down with your back to a chair with your knees apart, the weight of your body on your heels and your hands gripping the chair-seat behind you for support.

● push down on your hands so that you raise your pelvis and lift your chin upwards towards the ceiling, without arching your back too much — feel your thigh and pelvic muscles contracting
● return to the starting position; exhale
● repeat the exercise 10 times.

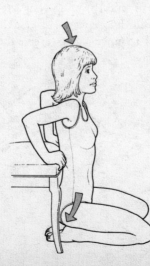

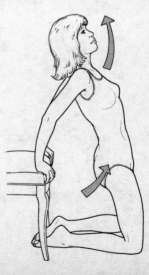

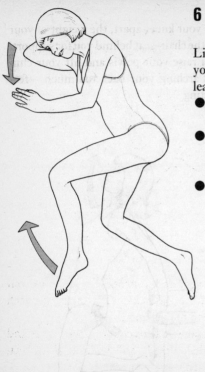

6   To improve respiration

Lie on your right side with your right arm folded and your right hand under your neck. Relax your left arm and left leg and lift them up in front of you, leaving your right leg bent and lying on the ground.

● simultaneously (a) stretch your left arm to the rear, and (b) stretch your left leg to the rear and inhale deeply

● simultaneously (a) bring your left arm forwards again, describing an arc above your head, and (b) bring your left leg forwards and downwards in an arc; exhale slowly

● after a series of 10 movements, reverse the procedure for the other side.

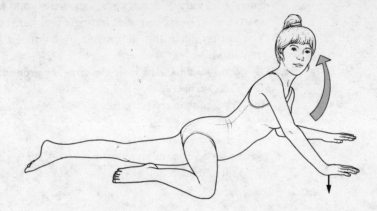

Lie on your stomach with your right leg bent and your left leg stretched out on the ground. Place your hands the width of your shoulders apart on each side of your head, and rest your left cheek on the ground.

- push down on your right hand so that you stretch your right arm and raise the right side of your body; inhale deeply and let your body turn slightly to lean on your left elbow, which is on the ground
- return to the ground by bending your arm; exhale
- after a series of 10 movements, reverse the procedure for the other side.

Lie on a bed with the back of your neck resting on the edge so that your head hangs backwards. Bend your legs with your knees together and your feet apart, and relax your arms, letting them hang downwards beside your head. You can reinforce this movement by holding a book weighing 1 or 2 kilos in your hands.

●   drop your hands a little closer to the ground; inhale

●   relax; exhale

●   repeat the exercise 10 times.

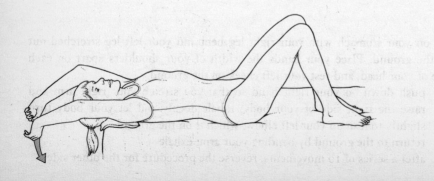

Sit down, with your hands at the back of your neck with your fingers interlocked and your legs together.

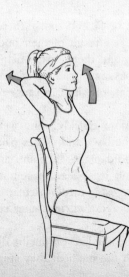

- take your elbows a little higher behind your head; inhale
- stretch your arms, turning the palms of your hands upwards; continue to inhale
- hold your breath in for a few moments
- bend your elbows and bring them in to squeeze your chest; exhale
- repeat the exercise 10 times.

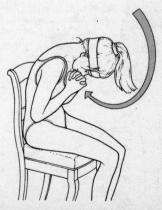

OBESITY AND UNDERWEIGHT

Obesity

OVERWEIGHT

reduced chest cavity

diaphragm abnormally high: reduced movement

distended digestive tract and abdomen

It is said that some people are quite happy to be fat. Of course there is some truth in this, but there are many who suffer as a result of their obesity, and the sarcastic quips they receive from those around them hardly help matters. Our modern age, so obsessed with good looks, is intolerant of overweight, regarding it as unaesthetic; but apart from that, obesity can cause numerous health problems.

Fat people get out of breath and tired more quickly. The weight of a large abdomen accentuates the curvature of the back and causes pains in the lumbar region. The extra weight carried around damages the joints and brings with it a real risk of arthritis in the back and legs. Serious conditions can ensue, for example hypertension, arteriosclerosis, cardiovascular illnesses, kidney disease and diabetes. Life expectancy is reduced (insurance companies take note!).

What is the answer? Fat people tend to try all the latest reducing diets, only to find that they start putting on weight again the moment they stop them –

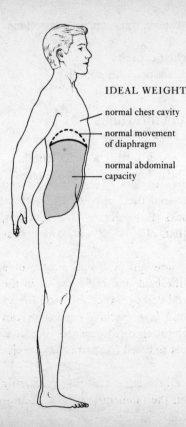

IDEAL WEIGHT

normal chest cavity

normal movement of diaphragm

normal abdominal capacity

and often add a few extra pounds to boot! Some seem destined to put on weight no matter how little they eat – it is this group who are the target of every 'miracle' slimming product selling campaign.

An average person has about 20 per cent body fat, while a very fat person has 50 per cent. How can this excess fat be got rid of? Is it to be a sauna, a sweat suit, or diuretics? It is unlikely that remedies of this sort will succeed in burning up excess fat – they merely result in fluid loss and put a strain on the kidneys, which then have to eliminate body wastes in a reduced volume of urine.

In an obese person the volume of the chest cavity is reduced by the distension of the abdomen, and the bottom of this thoracic cage keeps the abdomen in a state of tension, reducing the movement of the diaphragm, especially during exhalation. In moments of effort, the body's increased need for oxygen is not met, and it will obviously seek elsewhere the energy to compensate for this deficiency. The only possible solution seems to be an ever-greater demand for food. It is as though an obese person's body, unable to count on its respiratory factory, must have recourse to its digestive factory. Some overweight people have such great appetites that they eat without ever feeling that they have had enough: their stomachs and intestines are capable of distending to a considerable degree and will accept an astonishing volume of food.

A reasonable programme for losing weight, in addition to an appropriate diet, consists of:

● reduction of the storage capacity of the intestines, brought about by the

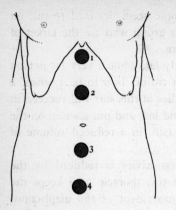

1 solar plexus
2 upper intestinal plexus
3 lower intestinal plexus
4 plexus of the lower abdomen

stimulation of the intestinal muscles and the nervous centres controlling them (reduction of 'food pockets')

● training in breathing to restore a suitable chest capacity
● regular physical exercise to replace the fatty tissues with muscle.

1   To reduce the storage capacity of the intestines

In all these abdominal exercises, pressure is applied with a quick rhythm (1 second of pressure on, 1 second of pressure off). This accelerates the transportation of material through the intestines.

Example: applying pressure to the solar plexus

Place your fingers under your sternum.

● apply pressure; exhale
● relax pressure; inhale
● repeat the procedure 10 times
● operate similarly on the other plexuses.

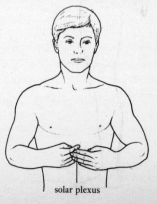

solar plexus

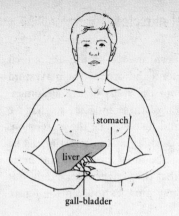

Hook your fingers under your right ribs.

- apply pressure and penetrate under your ribs; exhale
- relax the pressure and withdraw your fingers; inhale
- repeat the procedure 10 times.

This treatment involves your liver and gall-bladder in particular. Repeat the procedure under your left ribs, which involves your stomach.

To encourage the elimination of faeces

Place the fingers of one hand over those of the other above your right groin.

- apply pressure; exhale
- relax the pressure; inhale
- repeat the procedure.

Repeat along the path of your colon, on the points indicated in the illustration.

2 To strengthen the belt of abdominal muscles

A feature of obesity is the loss in tone and performance of the abdominal muscles. This allows the intestinal organs to distend and occupy the maximum volume, encountering only feeble resistance from the walls of the abdomen. We should try to improve the tone and function of these muscles so that we keep the intestines under the correct pressure and help reduce the distension. If we do this, we are also reducing the storage capacity of the intestines. The neglected transverse and oblique muscles of the abdomen are important here, because of the considerable abdominal surface that they cover. We should not forget that it is primarily the job of the transverse muscles to keep the figure trim.

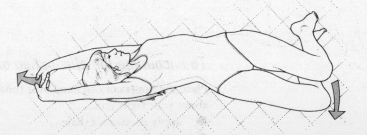

Lie on your back, with your fingers interlocked above your head and your legs relaxed and swung over to your right side.

- turn your head to the left and simultaneously (a) stretch your arms up above your head, and (b) stretch your thighs downwards by pushing your knees down – if necessary, push your feet against the floor to help; inhale
- return to the starting position; exhale
- after a series of 10 movements, reverse the procedure for the other side.

Lie on your back, with your left arm bent under your head and your right arm lying on the ground at right angles to your body.
- swing your left leg as far as possible across your right leg; exhale
- let your left leg spring back; inhale
- after a series of 10 movements, reverse the procedure for the other side.

3   To train respiration

The two previous stages are necessary for allowing respiration to function more freely. When the abdomen is distended its main muscle (the diaphragm) is prevented from rising and falling freely like a piston, while the inadequate

d muscles

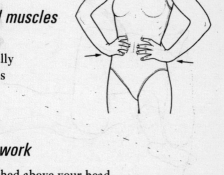

lly
s

work

hed above your head.

Exercise for the intercostal respiratory muscles

Sit down, fold your arms, and rest your elbows on the edge of a table. Turn your head to one side and rest it on your hands; place your buttocks well back in your seat.

- arch your back; inhale
- hollow your back; exhale fully
- continue exhaling forcibly for a few seconds
- repeat the exercise 10 times.

Exercise for the respiratory muscles at the top of the thorax

Entwine your fingers on top of your head.

- swell out the top of your chest and at the same time draw in your chin; inhale
- relax; exhale fully
- continue exhaling forcibly for a few seconds
- repeat the exercise 10 times.

Exercise for the whole of the respiratory system

Lie on your back on a bed with the upper part of your neck resting on the edge, and let your arms hang down relaxed over the side.

- stretch your body and lower your arms still further; inhale
- bring your bent and relaxed arms towards your abdomen; exhale fully
- continue exhaling forcibly for a few seconds
- repeat the exercise 10 times.

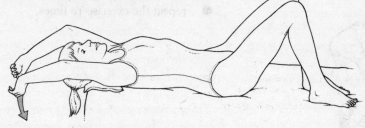

4   To improve kidney function

This exercise treats the autonomic nervous pathways connected with the functioning of the kidneys.

Place your left fist on your lower ribs, at the back. Press backwards so that you wedge your fist between your back and the back of the chair.

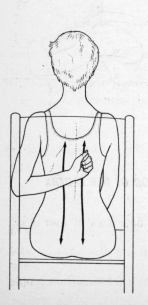

- lean backwards or press more strongly against the chair-back; inhale
- lessen the pressure by leaning slightly forwards; exhale; proceed in this way over the whole ridge of muscles in the bottom part of your back
- reverse the procedure for the other side.

Underweight

UNDERWEIGHT

— reduced chest cavity

— diaphragm abnormally low: reduced movement

— reduced abdominal capacity

An underweight person is usually made fun of less than a fat one, and most thin people, accustomed to being 'skinny' from infancy, are not bothered about it as long as they enjoy reasonable health. But there are some whose thinness makes them feel uncomfortable and somehow inferior.

Significant loss of weight can occur during a period of overwork, or as a result of an emotional or psychological upheaval. After such a loss people usually make every effort to regain their proper weight, although frequently the 'recovery phase' never comes to an end.

While a fat person seems to retain everything he eats, a thin one appears to retain nothing. He has a concave abdomen, a sunken rib cage, and his body seems to groan inside a prison. The slightest effort tends to leave him out of breath and decidedly tired. His stomach and intestines remain tight and incapable of retaining enough food for proper assimilation, resulting eventually in various forms of dietary deficiency. It is even possible for some thin people to consume a colossal volume of food without ever feeling that they've eaten enough, and without getting any fatter: they simply gain no benefit from their intake.

A reasonable programme for recovering one's proper weight, in addition to a reasonable and appropriate diet, consists of:

- improving the storage capacity of the intestines and the assimilation of nutrients, through gentle stimulation of the digestive tract and the nervous centres which control it
- improving respiration
- reducing any stress.

IDEAL WEIGHT

normal chest cavity

normal movement of diaphragm

normal abdominal capacity

1 To improve the storage capacity of the intestines

These exercises gently stimulate the digestive tract and the nervous centres controlling the muscular system of the intestines. Pressure should be applied with a slow rhythm to slow down the passage of material through your intestines and reduce the tightness in these organs.

- apply steadily increasing pressure for 5 seconds
- maintain the pressure for 5 seconds
- gradually reduce the pressure for 5 seconds.

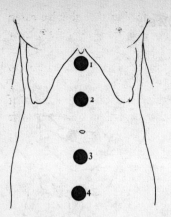

1 solar plexus
2 upper intestinal plexus
3 lower intestinal plexus
4 plexus of the lower abdomen

To put pressure on the plexuses

Place your fingers together under your sternum to locate your solar plexus.
- slowly apply pressure; exhale
- release the pressure; inhale
- repeat the treatment on your other plexuses.

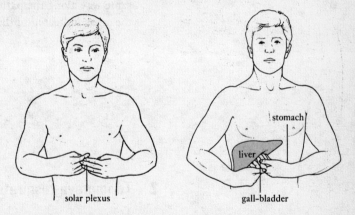

solar plexus

stomach
liver
gall-bladder

Hook your fingers under your right ribs.
- slowly apply pressure, penetrating underneath your ribs; exhale
- relax the pressure and withdraw your fingers; inhale.

This procedure involves your liver and gall-bladder in particular. Repeat the procedure under your left ribs, which involves your stomach.

To encourage regular emptying of the bowels

Place your fingers together above your groin.
- slowly apply pressure; exhale
- relax the pressure; inhale
- repeat the treatment 10 times. Proceed in the same way along the path of the colon on the areas indicated in the illustration.

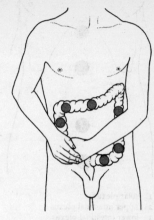

2   To improve respiration

Hyperactivity of the intestines holds the diaphragm down and prevents it moving freely. Inhalation in particular is difficult because of the lack of diaphragmatic tone. Treatment for underweight is the opposite to that for obesity, because we accentuate inhalation by holding the breath for between 5 and 10 seconds.

Exercise to assist total respiration

Lie on a bed with your neck resting on the edge and let your arms relax and hang over the side.

- stretch your body by letting your arms go lower still; inhale deeply
- hold your breath for a few seconds
- relax; exhale
- repeat the exercise 10 times.

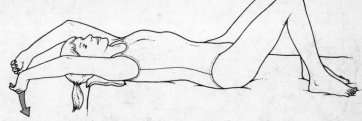

To relax the abdominal muscles which are often tensed up

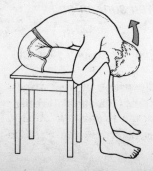

Sit down with your legs together, your abdomen against your thighs, your hands on your knees and your head hanging down.

- slowly inflate your abdomen; inhale deeply
- hold your breath for a few moments
- deflate your abdomen; exhale
- repeat the exercise 10 times.

Lie down on your back in a neutral position.

- slowly inflate your abdomen; inhale deeply
- hold your breath for a few moments then relax; exhale
- repeat the exercise 10 times.

To activate the diaphragm, which is very often sunken and without tone

Entwine your fingers, then place your hands on your head; put your legs together.

- stretch your arms up into the air, turning the palms of your hands upwards; inhale deeply and feel the base of your lungs (diaphragm) rising
- hold your breath for a few moments
- bring your hands down on to your head again; exhale
- repeat the exercise 10 times.

To exercise the intercostal muscles

Sit down with your arms folded and your elbows resting on the edge of a table; turn your head on one side resting on your hands, and position your buttocks well back on the chair.

- arch your back slowly and inhale deeply
- hold your breath for a few moments
- hollow your back; exhale
- repeat the exercise 10 times.

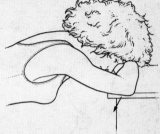

To exercise the respiratory muscles at the top of the chest

Entwine your fingers and rest them on the top of your head.

- swell out the top of your chest, drawing in your chin at the same time; inhale deeply
- hold your breath for a few seconds
- relax; exhale
- repeat the exercise 10 times.

3 To improve the blood supply to the back muscles

A good supply of blood to the back muscles helps to keep the back in good condition. It also reduces tiredness by allowing the rib cage to open more, thus improving the body's oxygen supply.

Sit on a chair and place your left fist on the right side of your spine under your shoulder-blade, then press back with your body to wedge your hand between your back and the back of the chair.
- lean backwards, or press more strongly against the chair-back; inhale
- hold your breath for a few seconds
- release the pressure by leaning slightly forwards; exhale.

Treat the ridge of muscles extending along the back to your buttocks in the same manner.
- reverse the procedure for the other side.

4 To relieve stress, See *Stress*, pp. 259–69.

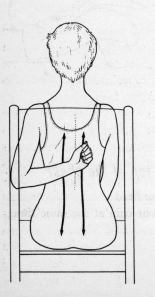

PAINS IN THE JOINTS AND MUSCLES
AS A RESULT OF AGEING

We all suffer at some time or another from aches and pains in the joints and muscles, but the most likely victims are those active in sports and people of advancing years: the former through intensive use of their bodies and the latter because they may have omitted, to their cost, to maintain their bodies in good order. The prospect of growing stooped and rickety haunts us all.

Growing old involves a lot of bodily changes: for example, losing flexibility and mobility, getting stiff and losing height, and suffering from inflamed tendons and joints. But aren't these also the symptoms that sporting enthusiasts complain of? Intensive training tends to shorten and contract muscles, and this imposes excessive pressure on the joints, leading to their deterioration. Conversely, a slowing down of life style causes the muscles to atrophy and become stiff; and joints that are not used gradually lose their mobility, just like a fractured limb imprisoned for some weeks in a plaster cast. The cartilagenous cells deteriorate and the ligaments harden. These examples illustrate an important principle of biology: anything which is not used atrophies and hardens, and what is over-used deteriorates.

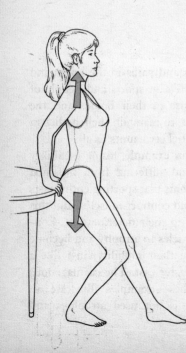

Are you old just because you've 'clocked up' a certain number of years? You only have to look around you to realize this is not so. There are young people who already look old, and there are old people who still look young. Our search for comfort and our frantic use of public and private transport deadens our muscles and their associated structures. Today we tend to be bombarded through the media by images of athletic healthy youth. But for a change, this chapter is addressed to everybody: to the potentially elderly who live in our technological civilization. We should not forget these two principles:

● our arm control starts with nerves issuing from the neck
● our legs are controlled by nerves issuing from the lumbar region.

Therefore, it is our neck and lumbar region that we should strengthen first. In this chapter the exercises concern only the limbs. Previous chapters have been devoted to the other parts of the body.

/ *The arms*

1 The shoulders

Stand with your back leaning against a desk or table, with the palms of your hands placed on the edge, your arms vertical and stretched, and your legs positioned to maintain your balance (partly bent, for example). The weight of your body is thus distributed more or less between your arms and your legs.

- sway over to your right side so that you bear most of your weight on your right arm; inhale; feel the stretching towards the top of your shoulder
- return to a central position; exhale
- sway over to your left side; inhale
- repeat the movements 10 times.

Stand with your left side 8–12 inches away from a wall; raise your left arm vertically and place the palm of your left hand on the wall as high as possible.
- slightly bend your left knee towards the wall and let your trunk lean the same way; inhale, and feel the stretching towards the base of your shoulder
- straighten your left knee; exhale
- after a series of 10 movements, reverse the procedure for the other side.

Hang by your hands from the top of a solidly fixed door (stand on a stool or on some books if the door is too high).
- gradually bend up your knees as far as you can while still feeling comfortable, while you hold on, bearing the weight of your body; inhale, and feel the stretching towards the base of your shoulders
- stretch your knees; exhale
- repeat the exercise 10 times.

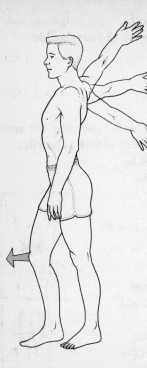

Stand with your right side about 20 inches away from a wall. Stretch your right arm horizontally backwards, place your right hand on the wall, and move your right foot forward.

- slightly bend your right knee; inhale, and feel the stretching in the back of your shoulder
- stretch your right knee; exhale
- repeat the procedure for the other side.

Stand facing a wall, then lean your hands on it the width of your shoulders apart. Your legs should be apart and straight, and far enough away from the wall for your back to be flat.

- drop your chest and feel your shoulders stretching; inhale
- let your chest spring up again; exhale
- repeat the movements 10 times.

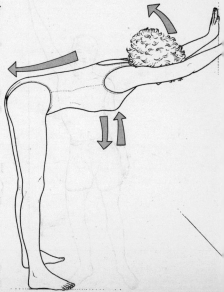

2   Elbows, wrists and hands

Kneel down on all fours, with the palms of your hands on the ground and your fingers turned backwards.

- pull your pelvis backwards; exhale, and feel your arms stretching right down to your wrists
- bring your pelvis forwards; inhale
- repeat the exercise 10 times.

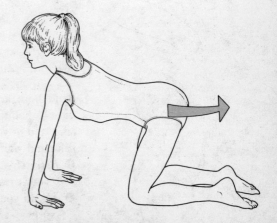

VARIATION: Standing, with your hands on the edge of a table.

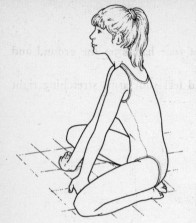

Kneel down and sit on your heels with your knees apart on the ground; place the palms of your hands between your knees, with your fingers pointing outwards and your arms straight.

- sway to the left; exhale, and feel your right arm stretching
- return to the central position; inhale
- sway to the right; exhale, and feel your left arm stretching
- repeat the exercise 10 times.

VARIATION: Do the same exercise standing up, with your hands on the edge of a table.

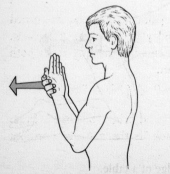

Bend both arms in front of you, with your hands back to back and your thumbs pointing forward. Take your right hand towards your left wrist as if to take hold of your left hand, then place the fingers of your right hand over your palm and your left thumb on the back of your right hand.

- stretch your elbows and take your hands horizontally outwards level with your eyes; exhale
- bend your elbows, and bring your hands back to your chest, reversing the previous movement; inhale
- after a series of 10 movements, reverse the procedure for the other side.

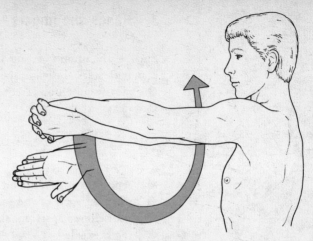

Stretch your arms out in front of you, with the palms of your hands turned outwards, your thumbs pointing downwards, and your hands back to back. Place your right hand over your left wrist and entwine the fingers of both hands, letting your right hand direct the movement.

- bend both elbows and bring your hands in an arc downwards and towards your face; inhale
- reversing the movement, stretch your elbows and bring your hands in an arc downwards and outwards to finish back in the starting position; exhale
- reverse the procedure for the other side.

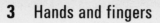

3   Hands and fingers

Encircle the thumb of your right hand with the fingers of your left hand; grip it on both sides at each of the interphalangial joints.
● move your elbows apart; inhale, and feel the joint stretching and loosening
● relax; exhale

● repeat the procedure on each of your fingers
● work on each of the joints with little twisting movements as you move your elbows apart; inhale
● relax; exhale.

Entwine the fingers of both hands in front of your chest, with your arms bent.
● stretch your arms in front of your eyes; exhale, and feel your wrists, hands, and fingers stretching
● bend your elbows and bring your hands back to your chest; inhale
● repeat the exercise 10 times
● repeat the exercise at different levels.

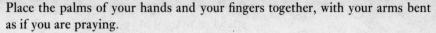

Place the palms of your hands and your fingers together, with your arms bent as if you are praying.

- bring both your hands vertically downwards together; exhale and feel your palms moving apart and your hands touching only at the tips of your fingers
- repeat the exercise 10 times.

VARIATION: Treat stiff fingers individually by performing the exercise with your other fingers bent out of the way.

// The legs

Place your knees on the floor the width of your shoulders apart so that your feet have their inside edge on the ground and your big toes touch the floor; stretch your arms in front of you.

- move your pelvis backwards; exhale, and feel the inside of your thighs stretching
- bring your pelvis forwards; inhale
- repeat the exercise 10 times.

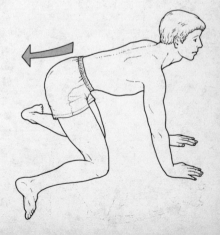

Go down on all fours with your legs stretched, your feet apart and your arms stretched in front of you.

- bend your right knee; exhale
- return to the starting position; inhale
- after a series of 10 movements, reverse the procedure for the other side.

SIMPLIFIED VARIATION: Stretch your arms out on to a stool.

Lie on your back with your right leg bent, your right foot on the ground, your left leg bent, and your left foot resting on your right knee. Place your hands on your left knee.

- push on your left knee with both hands; inhale, and feel the inside of your thigh stretching
- relax the pressure on your knee; exhale
- after a series of 10 movements, reverse the procedure for the other side.

Lie on your back with your right leg bent and resting on the ground. Place your left leg over your right leg, with your left hand under your neck and your right arm lying on the ground at right angles to your body.

● swing your left leg as far as possible to the right; exhale
● after a series of 10 movements, reverse the procedure for the other side.

Lie on your left side with your left hand under your neck, your right hand on the ground in front of you, and your legs folded over one another.

● swing your right leg backwards; inhale
● let your leg swing back; exhale
● after a series of 10 movements, reverse the procedure for the other side.

Lie on your stomach with your legs apart and your feet resting with their inner edges on the ground. Place your hands on the ground level with your face, and your chin on the ground.

- raise your chin gradually higher and higher; inhale, and feel the inside of your legs stretching
- bring your chin down to the ground; exhale
- repeat the exercise 10 times.

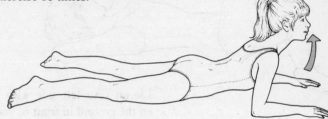

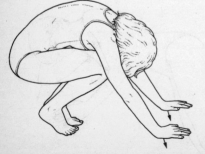

Crouch down with your arms stretched in front of you, your hands on the floor, and your buttocks against a wall.

- bring your pelvis down slightly to bring your heels to the floor; exhale, and feel your calves stretching
- let your heels spring back up; inhale
- repeat the exercise 10 times.

Kneel down with your left knee on the ground and the weight of your body resting on the heel of your left foot. Place your right knee on your left knee, with the upper side of your toes on the ground and your foot arched. Place your left hand on your hip or on the ground, with your right hand on the heel of your right foot.

● push slightly on the heel of your right foot with your right hand; exhale, and feel the upper part of your foot and leg stretching
● relax the pressure; inhale
● after a series of 10 movements, reverse the procedure for the other side.

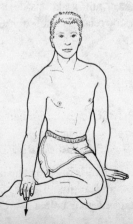

EXERCISES FOR STUDENTS

When we are studying we frequently find we are tensed up, with a backache or headache, after spending hours bent over books and notes, or staring at a VDU. Eventually we may reach a point where we feel we simply cannot take in any more. Is there anything we can do when our body refuses to go on? A few Wa-Do exercises can make us feel better and give us the energy to continue our studies or relax us ready for a restful sleep.

I *The head*

1 To relax the face

For the eyes and the muscles of the face

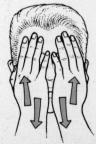

Rest the palms of your hands on your cheek-bones.
● close your eyes, and apply an even, constant pressure to your face using the whole surface of your palms

- operate upwards and downwards with small, regular movements, making the skin of your face and your eyelids slide over the underlying bone; breath steadily and naturally
- finish with gentle pressure from your palms on your closed eyes
- breathe calmly for a few moments.

For the side of the nose (sensitive after intense concentration)

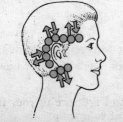

Gently pinch the bridge of your nose at its highest point, between your eyes.
- maintain a steady pressure, with your thumb on one side of your nose and your fingers on the other; keep your eyes closed
- operate with small, regular movements upwards and downwards, making your skin slide over the underlying bone; breathe naturally
- repeat the procedure along the length of the nose.

For the ears (sensitive after long hours of attentive listening)

With the three middle fingers of each hand, make small, regular movements which make your skin slide over the underlying bone.
- apply your fingers consecutively to the positions shown; breathe naturally.

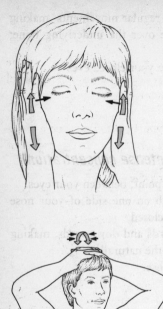

With the palms of your hands over your ears, maintain constant pressure; keep your eyes closed.

● operate with small, regular movements up and down, until you feel your ears getting warm.

Place the palms of your hands flat over your ears, with your fingers pointing backwards.

● accentuate the pressure on your ears; exhale
● relax the pressure slightly; inhale
● repeat the movements 10 times.

In this way you can induce a state of calm that is very beneficial after hours of listening, especially since the middle ear is one of the body's centres of balance.

2   To relax the scalp

Put your hands on the top of your head, with your fingers interlocked.

● lift your scalp by bringing the palms of your hands together; inhale
● relax; exhale
● repeat the procedure (a) along a central line running from the front to the back of your head, and (b) over the whole of your scalp.

3 To improve the blood supply to the head

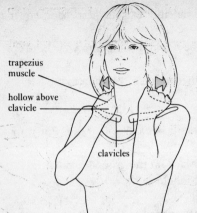

trapezius
muscle

hollow above
clavicle

clavicles

Our head needs a good supply of blood, for the areas mentioned in the preceding exercises, and also to relieve eye strain. Exercises repeated several times a day will prove beneficial to the nervous system and the brain.

Place your hands on each side of your neck and support your elbows on a table.
● keeping your head up straight, let your neck press against the palms of your hands; exhale, and feel the blood flowing into your face
● bring your neck slightly back while maintaining the same position; inhale
● repeat the movements 10 times
● operate in the same manner all along the neck.
(*Note:* these movements can be practised without support: it is enough to apply pressure with your palms while your hands point backwards.)

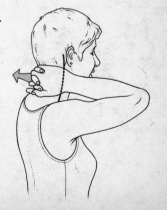

Place your hands over the back of your neck with your arms relaxed.
● raise the flesh and muscles of your neck by bringing your palms together; exhale
● relax slightly; inhale
● repeat the movement 10 times.

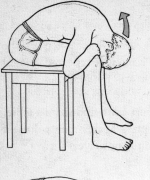

Place your knees apart with a hand on each one, and let your head hang down between your legs.

● let your head come up; exhale and feel the blood flowing into your head
● repeat the movement 10 times
● do the same again, lifting your head further to the right, then to the left.

Kneel down and place your hands on the ground beyond your head. Put your forehead on the ground.

● raise your hips and let your head roll forward on the ground; exhale
● bring your pelvis down on to your heels; inhale
● repeat the exercise 10 times
● repeat the exercise with your head slightly turned to the right, then to the left.

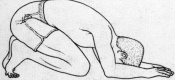

Lie on your back and raise your pelvis with the help of your hands and elbows; maintain the position.

● swell out your abdomen to inhale
● relax your abdomen to exhale
● repeat the exercise 10 times
● repeat the exercise, with your head slightly turned to the right, then to the left.

Lie on your back with your knees bent together and your feet apart on the ground, and your arms behind your head with the palms of your hands placed beside your ears. Point your fingers towards your feet, and push down on your arms so that the crown of your head comes into contact with the ground. Hold the 'bridging' position, without putting too much strain on your neck.

- push lightly on your feet so that you rock forwards on your head; inhale
- relax the pushing from your feet; exhale
- repeat the exercise 10 times
- bring your body down to the ground again by gently lowering first your head then the rest of your body.

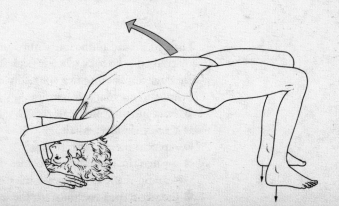

// *The neck and the arms*

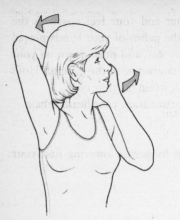

Turn your head to the left with your chin raised. Place your left hand under your chin with your right hand on your left temple.

● slightly exaggerate your head rotation; exhale
● relax slightly; inhale
● when the movement becomes easy at its furthest point, gradually increase your rotation span
● reverse the procedure for the other side.

Turn your head to the left with your chin lowered and the back of your neck stretched. Put your left hand under your chin and your right hand on your left temple.

● accentuate your head rotation; exhale
● relax slightly; inhale
● repeat the exercise 10 times
● when the movement becomes easy at its furthest point, gradually increase the extent of the rotation
● reverse the procedure for the other side.

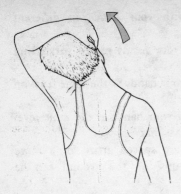

Incline your head to the right and curl your left arm over your head so that your left hand covers your right ear.

- accentuate your head movement by bringing your head down to your left shoulder with your left hand; exhale
- relax slightly; inhale
- repeat the exercise 10 times
- gradually increase the extent of the movement
- reverse the procedure for the other side.

'Press-ups' against the wall

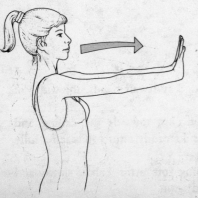

Face a wall at an arm's distance, then stretch your arms out in front of you with the palms of your hands on the wall, your shoulders' width apart. Point your fingers upwards; stretch your legs and place your feet apart.

- bend your elbows and take the weight of your body on your hands while your body stays quite straight; inhale
- push on your hands and stretch your arms to return to the starting position; exhale
- repeat the exercise 10 times.

You can increase your distance from the wall to give the muscles and joints of your arms more work.

The previous exercise can be performed with your hands in different positions.

- with your fingers pointing upwards, and your hands placed parallel on the wall at varying heights
- with your fingers pointing outwards, and your hands at the same level on the wall at varying heights
- with your fingers pointing downwards and your hands at the same level on the wall, and at the same height as your abdomen.

You can also vary the distance your hands are spaced apart for a more complete but more difficult exercise. 'Press-ups' on the ground can be practised too, but after the other variations.

/// *The trunk*

1 The back and the chest

Lie on your front with your chin on the ground and your hands, the width of your shoulders apart, level with your ears.

- gradually raise your body, lifting your chin towards the ceiling and straightening your arms; inhale slowly and steadily until you reach a fully stretched position
- gradually return to the ground by bending your arms; exhale slowly and steadily until you are lying on the ground again.

Lie on your front and take hold of your ankles; rest one cheek or your chin on the ground.
- push on your ankles as though to stretch your arms; inhale, and feel your body stretching like a bow and your chest being raised off the ground
- stop pushing on your ankles and let your chest sink down again; exhale
- repeat the exercise 10 times.
- if possible, roll backwards and forwards.

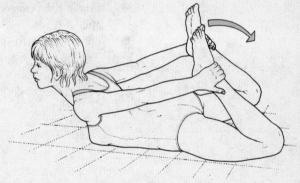

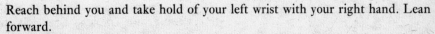

Reach behind you and take hold of your left wrist with your right hand. Lean forward.
- stretch both arms, and at the same time raise your chin; inhale
- relax; exhale
- repeat the exercise 10 times.

Lie on the ground with your left arm bent at an angle of 90 degrees, the fingers of your left hand pointing upwards, and your right arm lying along your body. Turn your head to the left. Lift both legs and put them over your left shoulder; hold the position.

- try to touch the ground, first with your feet, then with your knees; exhale
- relax slightly; inhale
- repeat the exercise 10 times.
- reverse the position of the body and repeat the exercise 10 times for the other side
- if possible, perform the exercise rolling straight over backwards.

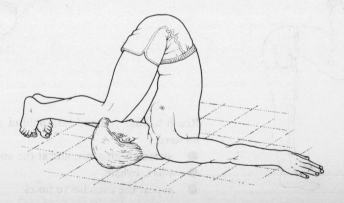

Place your hands at chest height on a wall, a piece of furniture or a door-frame; stand with your legs stretched and your feet apart so that your back is flat.

● lower your chest; inhale
● let it come up again; exhale
● repeat the exercise 10 times.

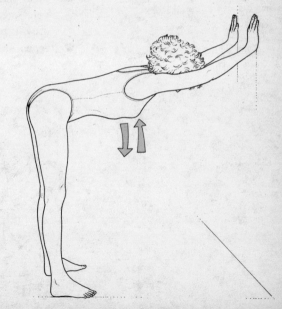

2   The abdomen and lumbar region

Sit towards the front edge of a chair with your hands on your knees.
- bring your knees up to your chest and push your head down towards your knees; exhale
- push your knees down and place your feet on the ground, then push on your knees with your hands so as to stretch your arms and the upper part of your body; inhale
- repeat the exercise 10 times.

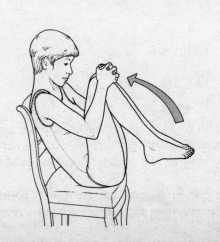
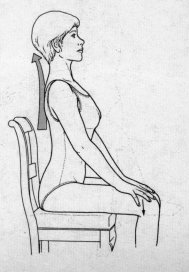

Sit on a chair and cross your left thigh over your right leg;
place your right hand on the outside of your left thigh,
with your other hand on the chair.
- push your left thigh towards the right with your
  right hand; exhale, and feel your trunk rotating
  above your legs
- stop pushing; inhale
- after repeating the exercise 10 times, reverse the
  procedure for the other side.

Stand with your left leg slightly behind your right.
- move your left leg quickly upwards towards the right as though kicking a
  football; exhale, and feel your arms swinging to the left to maintain
  balance
- let your left leg return to the starting position; inhale
- after repeating the exercise 10 times, reverse the procedure for the other
  side.

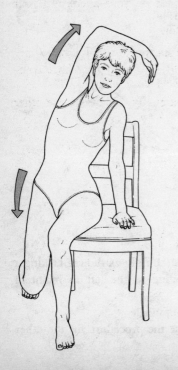

Sit on the edge of a chair with your left buttock on the seat and the right one off it; raise your right arm above your head, and put your left hand on the seat.

● simultaneously (a) let the weight of your body come on to your right buttock, which is lowered at the side of the chair, and (b) stretch your right arm as much as possible to the left; exhale

● after repeating the exercise 10 times, reverse the procedure for the other side.

IV   *The legs*

Stand with your legs wide apart, with your hands on your knees and your
arms stretched.

- half bend your right knee; exhale
- straighten your knee again and return to the starting position; inhale
- when you can do the exercise quite comfortably, bend your knee completely and lower yourself down on it
- after repeating the exercise 10 times, reverse the procedure for the other side.

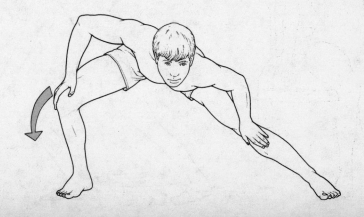

Stand with your hands apart, resting on a piece of furniture, your left knee bent and your right leg stretched well behind you.

- jump to reverse the position of the legs, bringing the right leg to the front with the right knee bent, and the left foot to the back with the left leg straight; inhale as you jump, exhale when you land
- repeat the exercise 10 times.

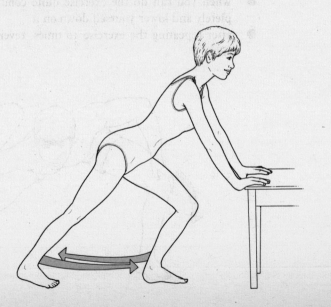

Stand with your hands on the knees and your feet together.

- bend your knees slightly and rotate them with a small circular movement, keeping your feet and your pelvis in the same position; inhale during one rotation, exhale during the next
- repeat the exercise 10 times, then rotate the knees in the opposite direction.

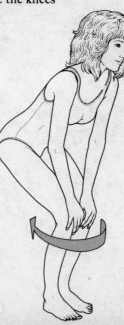

Conclusion

I hope that through this book you will find pleasure in living in harmony with your body, inhabiting it more comfortably, feeling *really good* deep down inside.

Your body is as precious to your life style as everything outside it. Don't ignore it – preserve its uniqueness. Instinct, common sense and regular attention can keep it healthy and happy. Follow Wa-Do and you'll make your body your *friend*, the sort of friend you like to have close at hand to help you and to surprise you.

If I've succeeded in interesting you in yourself and in motivating you to do something with yourself, then I shall be more than happy.

USE WA-DO TO FEEL GOOD!

3.95